diabetes

BREAKTHROUGHS

2012

diabetes
BREAKTHROUGHS
2012

Take Control—for Your Health, for Your Life

FROM THE EDITORS OF **Prevention**

RODALE

This book is intended as a reference volume only, not as a medical manual. The information given here is designed to help you make informed decisions about your health. It is not intended as a substitute for any treatment that may have been prescribed by your doctor. If you suspect that you have a medical problem, we urge you to seek competent medical help.

Mention of specific companies, organizations, or authorities in this book does not imply endorsement by the author or publisher, nor does mention of specific companies, organizations, or authorities imply that they endorse this book, its author, or the publisher.

Internet addresses and telephone numbers given in this book were accurate at the time it went to press.

Prevention is a registered trademark of Rodale Inc.

Printed in the United States of America

Rodale Inc. makes every effort to use acid-free ♾, recycled paper ♻.

Photo credits are on page 356.

ISBN-13 978–1–60961–793–6   hardcover

2   4   6   8   10   9   7   5   3   1   hardcover

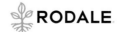

We inspire and enable people to improve their lives and the world around them.
For more of our products, visit **prevention.com** or call 800-848-4735.

To the millions of people
living with diabetes

CONTENTS

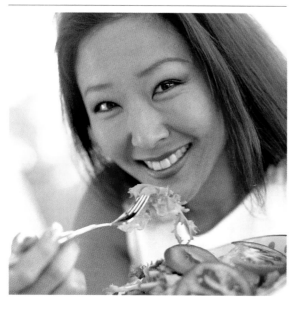 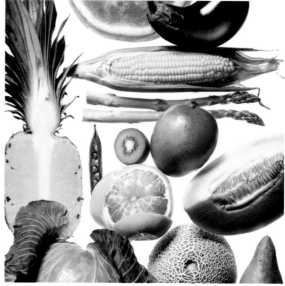

PART

1

TAKE CONTROL

PART

2

EAT RIGHT

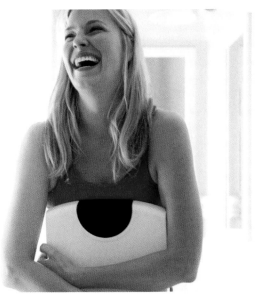

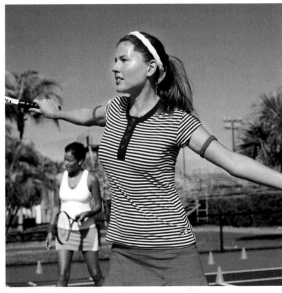

PART

3

LOSE WEIGHT

PART

4

MOVE IT!

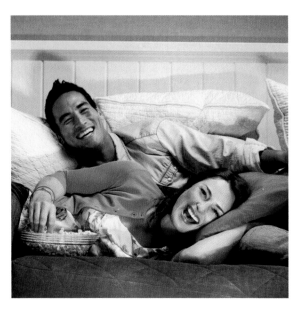

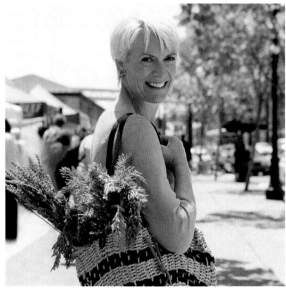

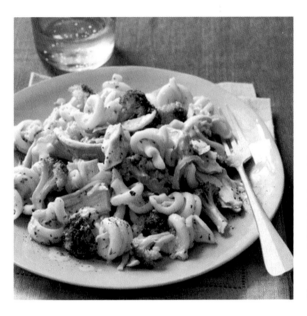

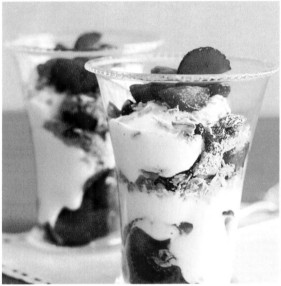

INTRODUCTION

Seven: That's the number of millions of Americans with undiagnosed diabetes. Although as you're holding this book in your hands, there's a good chance you're not one of them—that either you or someone you love has been diagnosed with diabetes.

What you do next is completely up to you. You can let that news derail your life, or you can let it bring your life into focus. Now you have a very important goal: to take control of your blood sugar. This book is filled with tips to help you do just that.

Part 1 will help you to "Take Control." You'll learn why blood sugar matters so much, the benefits of keeping your blood sugar in balance, and the tests that are crucial to managing your diabetes.

In Part 2, you'll find out how to "Eat Right." You'll discover the very best foods for people with diabetes. And you'll also find one key ingredient to avoid. You'll learn how to eat smarter, and safer, and consider taking supplements.

Part 3 tells why it's so important to "Lose Weight." Ninety percent of people who've been diagnosed with diabetes are overweight. Here you'll read smart food and weight-loss strategies to help you to lose weight, perhaps without even trying.

You'll "Move It" more after reading Part 4. Exercise can be very beneficial for everyone, but especially for everyone with diabetes. In this section you'll find lots of ways to work out, and even ways to make exercise fun as well as rewarding.

In Part 5, you'll read about the connection between mind and body in "Mind Matters." Stress isn't helpful when you have diabetes, so here you'll learn stress busters and stay-calm solutions. You'll also read about the restorative, healing powers of sleep.

Part 6 discusses the many complications of diabetes so this section will help you "Avoid Complications." Here you'll learn how to prevent some of the most common diabetes complications, including high blood pressure, heart disease, cancer, and even Alzheimer's disease.

You'll get cooking in Part 7 with our "Diabetes Cookbook." Here you'll find *Prevention*'s 100 best diabetes-friendly recipes. Some of our favorites are Double Pumpkin Snack Bars (see page 230), African Peanut Soup (see page 275), Broccoli and Cheddar Bake (see page 288), Instant Teriyaki Chicken (see page 308), and Walnut-Pumpkin Cheesecake (see page 347). We love them, and we hope you do, too.

Even though finding out you have diabetes can change your life, you *can* take control—for your health, for your life.

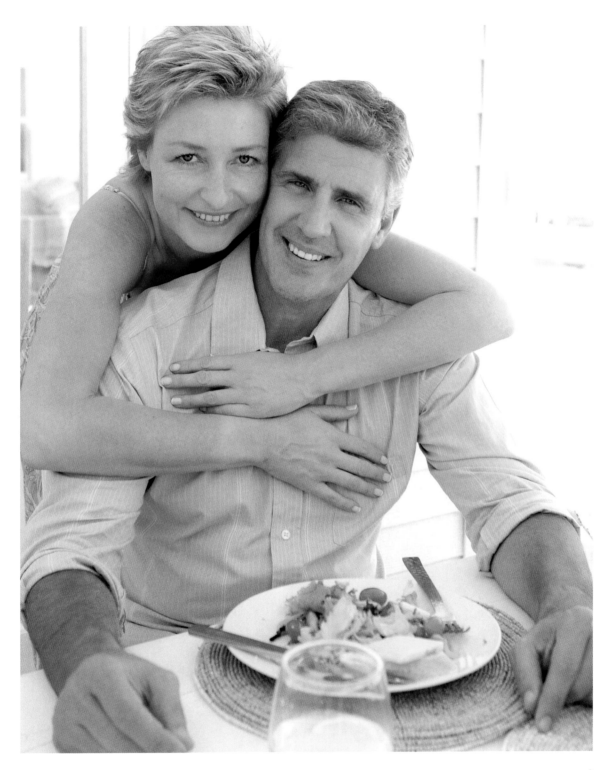

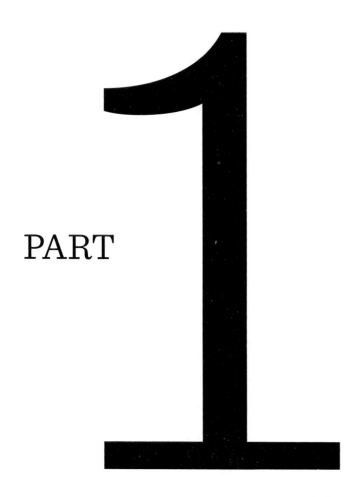

PART

1

TAKE

Knowledge is power, and here's the newest

CONTROL

research on diabetes to take back your life.

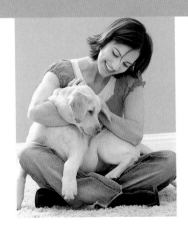 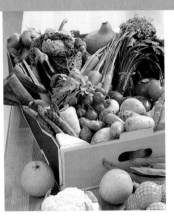 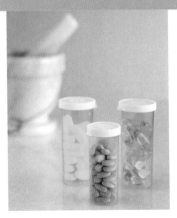

DIAGNOSTIC
Medical Breakthroughs

If you have received a diagnosis like diabetes, learning as much as you can about it can give you a sense of control. Information is power, and knowledge offers comfort. Here is the latest research about diabetes diagnostics to help you take charge of your health.

CONSIDER A DIABETES DOG

Diabetes used to rule Pebbles Miller's life. First diagnosed with type 1 diabetes as a teen, the 44-year-old mom from Antioch, California, had developed a condition that made her body insensitive to the warning signs of a dangerous drop in blood sugar. Even with monitoring and a healthy lifestyle, she suffered three strokes when her glucose levels unexpectedly plummeted.

But she recently got control of her disease, thanks to a 3-year-old yellow Labrador retriever named Fairmont. Now when Miller's blood sugar dips, Fairmont literally gets wind of it first. He's trained to pick up the scent of a chemical reaction that occurs in the body as blood sugar starts to drop. And when he does, he brings Miller a stuffed toy, which is a signal that she must take appropriate measures.

Diabetic service dogs are a new option for people with insulin-dependent type 1 or type 2 diabetes. Nonprofit organizations such as Dogs 4 Diabetics, Can Do Canines, and Canine Partners for Life provide their dogs for free or for a nominal donation. Diabetic Alert Dog charges up to $12,000, but they will also try to train an existing pet. After all, sometimes the best solution is right under your (dog's) nose.

BRING YOUR MEDS

Patients who bring their own medications with them to the hospital are half as likely to experience drug-related medical errors as people who forget them, a recent Australian study found. The most common mistake: People didn't get necessary meds, such as insulin or blood thinners, for preexisting health conditions.

CUT YOUR DRUG COSTS

Ask your doctor if he can prescribe a pill at twice the dose, to be cut in half by you or your pharmacist, reducing the cost by 50 percent. Also, fill your prescription at chain stores that sponsor savings programs for steep discounts. Walmart offers hundreds of $4 prescriptions. The Prescription Savings Club at Walgreens includes more than 400 generics priced at less than $1 a week.

AVOID CHEMICALS IN YOUR CANS

Canned food alert: *Consumer Reports* found bisphenol A—a chemical linked to diabetes, and also reproductive problems and heart disease—in all 19 brand-name canned foods it tested, including those labeled "BPA free." Because levels vary so widely, even among cans of the same product, there's no way to predict how much you're getting.

To reduce your risk, opt for frozen fruits and vegetables and for beans and tuna sealed in plastic containers, bags, or pouches, or use fresh ingredients whenever possible to make homemade soups, stews, and sauces.

■ TAKE THIS DIABETES TEST

How fast do you fall asleep?

If you routinely conk out in less than 5 minutes, that's a sign you're sleep deprived, says sleep expert Michael J. Breus, PhD. Skimping on sleep is linked to a host of serious ills, including diabetes, and also high blood pressure and weight gain. Sleep 30 minutes longer and see how you feel.

■ HEED THIS CLUE

If you snore every night and you're overweight, see your doctor. A study of almost 70,000 nurses found that those who sawed wood regularly had more than twice the normal risk of developing type 2 diabetes, regardless of their weight.

Regular deep snoring triggers the release of catecholamines, hormones that can promote insulin resistance, notes researcher Wael K. al-Delaimy, MD, PhD, of the Harvard School of Public Health. Sleep apnea, a condition in which you actually stop breathing numerous times a night, may have the same effect, he says.

■ DIAL UP FREE HEALTH ADVICE

You just burned your hand on a pan, and the doctor's office is closed. Now what? You could sit in the ER indefinitely or search online for advice, but here's another option: Call your insurance company. Many of them offer free 24-hour phone access to registered nurses who can advise about basic medical situations.

When *Prevention* staffers road-tested three of these services, RNs gave consistent advice that checked out when we followed up with doctors.

"Nurse hotlines are a great resource for nonurgent questions," says Sandra Schneider, MD, president of the American College of Emergency Physicians. If you have serious symptoms such as chest pain or a broken bone, however, you should call 911.

1

Why Blood Sugar

MATTERS

Americans are having a "sweet" crisis. Diabetes is an epidemic, with tragic consequences. But all you need to do is take charge of your blood sugar. Here's why—and how.

Imagine pouring a 5-pound bag of sugar down your throat. Absurd, right? Wrong. New research shows that this is how much sugar each American man, woman, and child gets each month—and most of it doesn't come from the sugar bowl. Sweeteners go by more than 50 names and hide out in virtually all processed foods, from your morning doughnut to those lunchtime baked beans, from fruit-flavored yogurt to the ketchup on your burger.

Added sugars in the American diet have grown exponentially since the early 1900s—by more than 2,100 percent—adding calories and edging out more nutritious fare. Researchers say it's no coincidence that as the food we eat grows sweeter, rates of overweight and blood sugar problems—including insulin resistance, metabolic syndrome, prediabetes, full-blown type 2 diabetes, and even pregnancy diabetes—have soared.

Sugar entwines us in a love-hate relationship. Your body needs a steady supply of blood sugar, the primary fuel burned by your cells. It plays a central role in physical and mental well-being. Your brain, for example, runs almost entirely on blood sugar (glucose). Your muscles can burn fat in a pinch, but they prefer blood sugar for zip. A baby growing in a mother's womb relies on it, too.

But the carbohydrates we eat and drink—the source of virtually all blood sugar—are more treacherous than ever before. Refined carbs (white bread, cakes, and snack foods) can make blood sugar skyrocket to dangerous levels. There's also growing evidence that high-fructose corn syrup (HFCS), now the most ubiquitous sweetener in the American food supply, is directly linked to the nation's twin epidemics of overweight and diabetes.

HFCS's role? This sweetener seems to bypass the body's "I feel full" mechanisms. In a study of 93,000 women, Harvard School of Public Health researchers recently linked a 10-pound weight gain and 83 percent higher diabetes risk directly to the consumption of HFCS.

Add other 21st-century factors that also pack on pounds and disrupt blood sugar levels—including big portions, fatty fast foods, and inactivity—and you've got a blood sugar crisis. Up to half of Americans have a prediabetic condition called insulin resistance, which is a serious early-stage blood sugar control problem that won't even show up on a blood sugar test. As many as 79 million have prediabetes (above-normal blood sugar levels), and 25.8 million have full-blown type 2 diabetes. Meanwhile, the number of children and teens with type 2 diabetes has increased six- to tenfold since 1994, mirroring the childhood obesity epidemic.

The bottom line for you: Blood sugar problems can zap your energy levels, make weight loss difficult or nearly impossible, and put you at risk for an astonishing variety of serious health problems, including heart attack, stroke, Alzheimer's disease, some cancers, infertility, blindness, kidney failure, amputation, and sexual difficulties. And that's not sweet.

Prehistoric Bodies, Drive-Thru Lifestyles

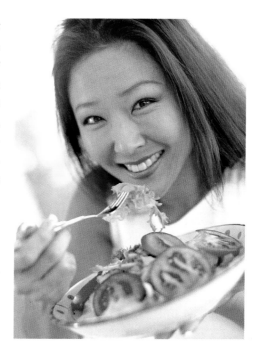

"Our bodies are essentially the same as they were 40,000 years ago, but our eating and exercise habits have changed tremendously," says Bryant Stamford, PhD, director of the Health Promotion and Wellness Center at the University of Louisville in Kentucky. "The same number of calories it might have taken our prehistoric ancestors an entire day to hunt and gather we can now have brought to our door with a phone call. We simply eat too much and exercise too little."

The tips in this book can help you bring your lifestyle back into harmony with your body's true needs. Through healthy eating, weight loss, and exercise, you can support your blood sugar control system, reducing your blood sugar and dampening elevated levels of insulin, a key blood sugar control hormone. The advantage: You can step off the sugar "spike and dip" roller coaster that contributes to stubborn weight gain, fatigue, moodiness, and cravings. You'll protect yourself against the profoundly damaging effects of high insulin and high blood sugar. You'll feel more energetic.

Seven Benefits of Balance

Our quiz on page 14 can help you size up your risk. But first, check out these compelling benefits of lowering and balancing your blood sugar.

Easier weight loss—without food cravings. If your blood sugar control system is out of whack, high levels of insulin might slow your body's fat-burning ability even on a low-calorie diet. Low blood sugar levels—the result of insulin doing its job too well—can trigger food cravings. You're stuck in a cycle of overeating and weight gain.

Bringing blood sugar and insulin down to healthier levels can stop cravings that prompt you to reach for another cookie at 3:00 p.m. or another handful of chips while you watch Jay or Conan or Dave late at night. As Tufts University researchers discovered in a recent study, it helps overweight people with high insulin levels lose more weight, perhaps by allowing fat cells to release their stores so that the body can burn them at last.

Energy to burn. What you eat affects your energy levels as well as your weight. Overeating high-glycemic carbs such as white bread, sweet snacks, and sugary

DOC, HOW'S MY BLOOD SUGAR?

We encourage you to call your doctor soon to schedule a fasting blood sugar test, one of the easiest in-office screenings (and one that's covered by most insurance plans). Far too many Americans live with undiagnosed type 2 diabetes and unrecognized prediabetes—uncontrolled high blood sugar that accelerates your chances of serious, life-threatening complications. Here's what you need to know.

TEST AS SOON AS POSSIBLE IF YOU HAVE ANY OF THE FOLLOWING RISK FACTORS FOR TYPE 2 DIABETES

- Family history of type 2 diabetes
- Overweight
- History of diabetes during pregnancy (gestational diabetes) or having a baby weighing 9 pounds or more at birth
- Low HDL cholesterol level (under 50 for women, below 40 for men), high total cholesterol (above 200), or triglycerides above 150
- High blood pressure (over 130/85)
- Age over 45
- Inactive lifestyle
- African American, Latino, Asian, Native American, or Pacific Island ethnicity

CHOOSE THE BEST TEST FOR YOU

We recommend a fasting plasma glucose test for most people. For this check, you will first fast for 8 to 12 hours, then visit the doctor's office or a lab to have your blood drawn. Your blood sugar is normal if the result is 99 milligrams of glucose per deciliter of blood (mg/dl) or lower; prediabetic if your sugar level is between 100 and 125 mg/dl; or potentially diabetic if it's over 125 mg/dl. (Your doctor will likely retest on another day before diagnosing type 2 diabetes.)

If you are pregnant, experiencing infertility or miscarriage problems, or concerned about

drinks floods your bloodstream with sugar, triggering a corresponding flood of insulin to move it out of the blood. The result: low blood sugar, which causes fatigue. Switching to better-quality body fuel like fiber-rich fruits and vegetables and healthy fats will keep you alert and energized for hours.

Improved fertility. Polycystic ovary syndrome (PCOS), the leading cause of infertility among women, is a serious blood sugar control problem that involves insulin resistance (when cells ignore insulin's signals to absorb blood sugar) and high insulin levels, experts now know. (Research also shows that PCOS can

prediabetes despite a normal fasting check, your doctor will perform an oral glucose tolerance test. You'll fast, then drink a sugary concoction of 75 grams of glucose (100 grams for a pregnant woman). Blood is drawn before you drink and up to four times afterward. Prediabetes is indicated when readings after 2 hours are between 140 and 199 mg/dl. Readings of 200 mg/dl or higher are considered indicative of full-blown diabetes. You've got gestational diabetes if you have any two of these results: fasting blood sugar over 95 mg/dl; blood sugar of 180 mg/dl 1 hour after drinking the sugary beverage; 155 mg/dl after 2 hours; 140 mg/dl after 3 hours.

If you couldn't fast or weren't expecting a blood sugar check at your doctor's appointment, your doctor might perform a random plasma glucose test. This nonfasting check is the least sensitive blood sugar check; it can miss slightly elevated sugar levels, making it a poor choice for people concerned about prediabetes. Your blood sugar is considered normal if the result is 140 mg/dl or lower and diabetic at 200 mg/dl or higher. If you opt for this test, ask for a follow-up fasting check to confirm your results.

TEST IN THE MORNING

You're apt to get a truer picture of where your blood sugar stands if you get tested in the morning as opposed to the afternoon. This realization emerged when scientists from the National Institute of Diabetes and Digestive and Kidney Diseases compared results of fasting plasma glucose tests given to 12,800 people. Only half the people with morning levels high enough to qualify as diabetic would have been detected if their tests had been done in the afternoon.

AND TEST AGAIN

If your blood sugar is normal, your doctor will probably recommend rechecking it in 1 to 3 years. If you are at risk for diabetes, however, ask for annual rechecks to catch creeping sugar levels early, when lifestyle changes can do the most to control them. If you have prediabetes or diabetes, work with your doctor to create a plan to track and lower your levels.

occur with or without ovarian cysts.) High insulin prompts your ovaries to churn out male hormones that disrupt ovulation, wreak havoc with your skin and hair, lock stubborn fat at your waistline, and raise your risk for diabetes, heart disease, and some cancers. Keeping your blood sugar steady and improving your insulin sensitivity can help right the balance.

Slimmer, healthier kids. Inactivity, fast food, and a sugar- and fat-laden diet are big reasons that the number of overweight kids in America has doubled since 1980, and the number with type 2 diabetes has skyrocketed. In Part 4, we'll show you how to incorporate more activity into your family's day to further cut their risk for overweight and blood sugar problems.

Lower risk for devastating health problems. High levels of circulating blood sugar and insulin can damage virtually every cell and organ in the body, significantly raising your odds for heart attack, stroke, high blood pressure, type 2 diabetes, cancer, blindness, kidney failure, amputation, and more. Controlling your blood sugar with the lifestyle strategies described in this book can reduce your risk for these potential killers and complications.

A sharper memory. People who don't process blood sugar normally are likely to have memory problems and even shrinkage of the brain region crucial for recall. However, a healthy lifestyle can help shield your brain from age-related memory loss and perhaps protect against Alzheimer's disease.

A healthier pregnancy and baby. If you're considering having children, balancing your blood sugar with a healthy diet and regular physical activity can help you avoid pregnancy diabetes, thus lowering your risk for full-blown type 2 diabetes later in life. You'll also protect your baby from injury during delivery and from blood sugar problems of her own after birth. Following the advice in this book before pregnancy will cut your risk for this condition.

Lose Weight, Feel Great

Healthy eating is one of the cornerstones of blood sugar control. You'll find dozens of healthy, delicious recipes in this book. Healthy eating can be both tasty and satisfying.

Physical activity is also a critical factor in blood sugar balance. For example, building muscle helps the body use insulin more efficiently, which lowers your blood sugar and insulin levels, encourages weight loss, and cuts health risks. This book offers many ways to get moving, including walking and even running. Also, lifting weights has been proven to help lower blood sugar, and you'll find many terrific exercises in this book.

The third leg of blood sugar balance is adequate, restful sleep and stress reduction. Both too little sleep and too much stress raise levels of stress hormones that in turn raise blood sugar levels. In Part 5 of this book, we offer strategies to reduce stress and sleep better. A balanced life also requires the active pursuit of pleasure, not merely the avoidance of stress, so think about ways to add more healthy joy to your life.

As you start your journey toward better health, keep in mind all the benefits of managing your blood sugar. You'll have more energy. Lose a few pounds. Prevent the symptoms of elevated blood sugar that erode your quality of life, such as fatigue, lethargy, and mood swings. And that's just for now. In the long run, you'll lower your chances of getting diseases that can rob you of precious years and ensure that you always live at peak energy and health.

The Importance of Knowing Your Numbers

Don Werkstell's motto is "check, check, and recheck." A former Department of Homeland Security inspector, he made sure that cargo flying in and out of Terminal A at Dallas/Fort Worth International Airport posed no threats. Diagnosed with type 2 diabetes in 2004, he now applies the same "check and check again" philosophy to his own blood sugar.

"I have to know what my numbers are. It's the only way to keep my blood sugar low and avoid all the complications of diabetes," says Werkstell. "I check my blood sugar all the time and guide my exercise and food choices by it. And every few months, I get a long-term test called an A1c. Diabetes runs in my family. I've seen what can happen if you don't take care of yourself."

Most of the 25.8 million Americans with diabetes aren't as in control as Werkstell. Despite government-sponsored health campaigns and newspaper and TV headlines, most of us are still in diabetes denial.

■ One-third of all Americans with diabetes don't know they have it.

■ Among those who do, most are still in danger. In mid-2005, a stunning new survey of 157,000 diabetic women and men revealed that while 85 percent think they're keeping the lid on high blood sugar, two out of three actually have dangerously high levels that can lead to kidney failure, blindness, amputation, deadly heart attacks, and stroke. The survey was commissioned by the American Association of Clinical Endocrinologists.

■ When Harvard Medical School researchers recently checked up on diabetes care at 30 of the nation's top university medical centers, they uncovered shocking neglect. Half the time, people with diabetes were sent home without the medicines they needed to lower dangerously rising blood sugar, leaving them at unnecessary risk for complications.

What's gone wrong? People with diabetes —and their doctors—underestimate the urgent need to keep blood sugar tightly controlled through diet, exercise, stress reduction, regular blood sugar checks, and medication if necessary.

In fact, a University of California, Los Angeles, study underscores the power of diet for people with diabetes. In this small, controlled 3-week study, 6 of 13 overweight or obese men with type 2 diabetes finished diabetes free, with normal blood sugar levels. How? With meals that were low in fat (12 to 15 percent of calories), moderate in protein (12 to 25 percent), and high in carbs (65 to 70 percent). Participants also walked for 45 to 60 minutes a day. But eating low-fat foods and no refined carbs—absolutely no toaster pastries or brownies—was critical to their success, says researcher Christian Roberts, PhD, the author of the study. He predicts that sticking to the diet long term may undo heart damage associated with diabetes.

But if you've had diabetes for a few years, diet may not be enough.

"Every time you see your doctor about your diabetes, you should discuss how well your treatment plan is working and whether it needs to be changed," says Kenneth J. Snow, MD, acting chief of the Adult Diabetes Division at the Joslin Diabetes Center in Boston. "You can't judge your diabetes by the number of pills you take. You should gauge it by your blood sugar—and by how well your treatment plan mix of diet, exercise, and medication is working to keep it low."

Cutting-edge diabetes treatment calls for aggressive care, particularly for the millions of people whose diabetes developed earlier in life, says Anne Peters, MD, director of the University of Southern California's clinical diabetes program and author of *Conquering Diabetes: A Cutting-Edge, Comprehensive Program for Prevention and Treatment.* "If your doctor seems behind the curve, ask what's going on. This is especially important if you're in your thirties, forties, fifties, or even your sixties. If your diabetes is diagnosed when you're younger or if you plan on living a long life, there's less room for error. High blood sugar is more dangerous when it goes on for years and years."

If your blood sugar is higher than your target goal, your doctor should be talking about a revised treatment plan, Dr. Peters says. If he doesn't bring it up, you should.

Diabetes 101

You've got type 2 diabetes if your blood sugar is over 125 milligrams of glucose per deciliter of blood (mg/dl) on a fasting blood sugar test, or over 200 mg/dl on an oral glucose tolerance test (in which you fast, then consume a sugary beverage, and take a blood test 2 hours later). If your blood sugar has soared to these levels, it means that nearly every aspect of your body's blood sugar control system has been damaged at a cellular level.

Diabetes is the last stop in a decades-long series of breakdowns in that system. Here's how the progression from normal blood sugar to diabetes unfolds: Thanks to a powerful combination of genetics, overweight, inactivity, abdominal fat, and stress, cells throughout your body first become insulin resistant, ignoring this vital hormone's signals to absorb blood sugar. To compensate, beta cells in your pancreas crank out extra insulin. Finally, your beta cells wear out. Insulin production drops; blood sugar rises. At first, sugar levels are only slightly higher than normal, a condition called prediabetes. But finally, as more beta cells cease functioning, your blood sugar rises to officially diabetic levels.

Many people discover their diabetes only after years of undetected high blood sugar have led to outward symptoms. Fatigue, thirst, getting up frequently at night to use the bathroom, frequent infections and slow-healing wounds, sexual difficulties (such as vaginal dryness and erection problems), and digestion trouble (diarrhea, vomiting, and slow digestion, all resulting from nerve damage) are all warning signs of type 2 diabetes. If you have any of these problems, call your doctor and schedule a blood sugar test!

Once diagnosed, you're in a whole new world. Suddenly, you must learn to operate a blood sugar meter—and find room for it in your purse or briefcase and in your busy schedule. Meals morph into arithmetic problems if you're trying to control blood sugar by counting carbohydrate grams or exchanges. And the pills! You might take 1, 2, or even 10 to 15 medications to lower your blood sugar and protect against diabetes-related heart risks such as high blood pressure and high cholesterol. You need to worry about your feet (even the smallest bump or cut could lead to a major infection), your eyes (high blood sugar can lead to vision problems), your kidneys (excess blood sugar can lead to kidney failure), and more. Small wonder, then, that people with diabetes report feeling more stressed and depressed.

This book's healthy living strategies can help you feel in control again.

The Diabetes Breakthroughs: What's Your Risk?

Living with high blood sugar or a related blood sugar control problem is a lot like having termites in your home: Serious damage can happen well before you notice something's wrong. But caught in time, most high blood sugar can be corrected before lasting damage occurs.

While it's not always possible to prevent high blood sugar, there's a lot you can do to lower your risk. And if your blood sugar is already above normal or you have a prediabetic condition called metabolic syndrome, you can start taking steps to reduce your chances of suffering its serious and even life-threatening consequences, including full-blown diabetes, heart attack, stroke, infertility, blindness, kidney failure, amputation, and even dementia and cancer.

"No question: Our research shows that many blood sugar problems can be controlled through lifestyle factors such as diet and exercise, especially if people act early," says David M. Nathan, MD, director of the diabetes center at Massachusetts General Hospital in Boston and chairman of the National Institutes of Health Diabetes Prevention Program (DPP). The DPP—a landmark study that looked at the effects of diet and exercise, medication, or a placebo in 3,234 people with high-normal blood sugar—demonstrated just how powerful even small lifestyle changes can be. People in the study who lost just 7 percent of their body weight and exercised just half an hour most days of the week cut their risk for developing diabetes by an amazing 58 percent. In contrast, study volunteers who took medication cut their risk by a lower 31 percent.

Take the following quiz and find out if your lifestyle protects you from high blood sugar or raises your risk. When you're done, read the brief explanation accompanying each correct answer. You're on your way to living a better way—with lower blood sugar, a trimmer figure, and a healthier future.

1. **What do you usually eat for breakfast?**
   a. High-fiber, whole grain cereal or oatmeal with fresh fruit and fat-free milk
   b. Scrambled eggs and buttered toast
   c. Pastry and a cup of coffee

2. **You watch TV this often:**
   a. 1 hour a day
   b. 2 hours a day
   c. 2+ hours a day

3. **What type of milk do you use most often?**
   a. Fat-free
   b. 2% fat
   c. Regular

4. **You need to get to the third floor of a high-rise. Will you:**
   a. Take the stairs and consider it a mini workout
   b. Take the stairs but huff and puff a bit
   c. Take the elevator

5. **How much time do you spend each week on a physical activity that makes you sweat, such as walking or strenuous physical work?**
   a. At least 2½ hours a week
   b. About 1½ hours a week
   c. Usually zero minutes a week

6. **When you make toast or a sandwich, you use:**
   a. Whole grain or multigrain bread
   b. Rye bread
   c. White bread

7. You sauté veggies in:
   a. Olive oil
   b. Vegetable oil
   c. Butter

8. You lift weights or do some other type of resistance training (resistance bands, weight machines):
   a. At least twice a week
   b. Less than twice a week
   c. Never

9. Which best describes your ability to handle stress?
   a. Most of the time, I can stay calm and productive despite stress.
   b. I lose my cool once in a while.
   c. I become tense and anxious the minute things don't go as expected.

10. How often do you eat beans?
    a. Frequently—at least five times a week
    b. Fairly often—once or twice a week
    c. Rarely, if ever

11. Do you smoke cigarettes?
    a. No
    b. A few a day
    c. Ten or more a day

12. How often do you eat each day (including snacks), and how large are those meals?
    a. Three moderate meals and several small snacks
    b. Three square meals a day
    c. I skip meals and usually have one or two big meals only

13. What's your alcoholic beverage of choice?
    a. Don't drink
    b. Wine
    c. A mixed drink or beer

14. How many hours of sleep do you usually get at night?
    a. $7\frac{1}{2}$ hours or more
    b. Between 6 and $7\frac{1}{2}$ hours
    c. Fewer than 6 hours

15. If you've had a fasting blood sugar test in the past year, the test result was:
    a. Under 100 mg/dl
    b. 100 to 125 mg/dl
    c. 126 mg/dl or higher

16. My cholesterol, triglycerides, and/or blood pressure are:
    a. At healthy levels
    b. Just a little out of whack—my blood pressure is slightly higher than 130/85, my triglycerides are a bit over 150 mg/dl, and/or my "good" HDL is below 50 mg/dl (for women) or below 40 mg/dl (for men)
    c. In the danger zone—my doctor has told me that my total cholesterol is over 200, my "bad" LDL is above 130 (or above 100 for people with diabetes or heart disease), my HDL is below 50 (for women) or 40 (for men), and/or my blood pressure is above 130/85

17. Grab a tape measure and measure your waist. The result is:
    a. Less than 35 inches if you're a woman or 40 inches if you're a man
    b. 35 inches or more if you're a woman
    c. 40 inches or more if you're a man

SCORING

Give yourself 3 points for every "a," 2 for every "b," and 1 for every "c."

From 51 to 41 points. Way to go! You're doing a great job helping your body process its blood sugar properly.

From 40 to 36 points. Nice work! You'll need to make just a few changes, especially if you're overweight or have other risk factors for high blood sugar.

From 35 to 31 points. Careful! This score puts you close to the danger zone, particularly if you have any of the risk factors for high blood sugar.

If you scored 30 points or lower. Uh-oh! Call your doctor, who can test your blood sugar and recommend lifestyle changes.

ASSESS YOUR SCORE

The best answer to every question is "a." Here's why.

1. Reach for fiber. Research shows that foods high in fiber, especially the soluble fiber in oatmeal, slow the absorption of glucose—the sugar molecules that fuel every cell in your body—into the bloodstream, which helps control blood sugar levels.

2. Move to lower blood sugar. Moderate exercise keeps muscle cells sensitive to insulin, the hormone that helps usher blood sugar into cells. Being an inactive couch potato makes your cells resist insulin, so blood sugar has trouble getting inside them, raising your risk for diabetes, cardiovascular disease, and stubborn overweight. The best fitness plan? A combination of walking or another calorie-burning aerobic exercise such as swimming or an exercise class, easy strength training, and plenty of everyday activity.

3. Sip diabetes-preventing milk. Even if you're overweight, consuming more low-fat dairy products, such as fat-free milk, could help reduce your risk of insulin resistance. In a 10-year study of 3,000 people, those who were overweight but got lots of dairy foods were 70 percent less likely to develop insulin resistance than those who avoided dairy. Milk sugar (lactose) is converted to blood sugar relatively slowly, which is good for blood sugar control and reducing insulin levels. Nutrients in dairy products (choose low-fat or fat-free varieties), including calcium, magnesium, and potassium, also help.

4. Find fitness opportunities everywhere. Climbing stairs burns extra calories and gives the heart a workout. It's one small way to help head off blood sugar problems that result from inactivity and overweight.

5. Activate the 30-minute exercise solution. Exercising at a moderate intensity (walking briskly, for example) for just 30 minutes a day, 5 days a week, can reduce the risk of developing type 2 diabetes by 58 to 80 percent. Exercise is most protective if you also adopt a healthy diet. People who don't exercise at all increase their risk by 25 percent.

6. Choose low-glycemic grains. Whole grain bread is higher in fiber, which helps slow the rate at which sugar enters the bloodstream. Fiber also helps you maintain a healthy weight. To make sure you're getting whole grain wheat, for example, look for the words "100 percent stone-ground whole wheat" on the ingredients list and for at least 3 grams of fiber per slice.

7. Say yes to good fats. Olive oil and other good sources of monounsaturated fat, such as flaxseed oil, avocados, and nuts, might help lower your risk for blood sugar problems and related cardiovascular conditions.

8. Build sleek, sexy muscle. Resistance training builds muscle density—stronger muscles that use more glucose. Along with aerobic exercise, it also aids weight loss.

9. Ease anxiety. Chronic stress increases the risk for high blood sugar several ways: Stress hormones trigger the release of extra blood sugar and also direct the body to store more fat in the abdomen, which raises your risk for insulin resistance and, ultimately, diabetes. Consider great stress-reducing strategies, such as yoga, deep breathing, and knitting.

10. Open a can of beans. Whether they're kidney, pinto, black, or white, beans are packed with soluble fiber, which blunts the entry of glucose into the bloodstream. Soluble fiber also helps lower bad LDL as well as homocysteine, a compound in the blood associated with heart disease.

11. Make your life a no-smoking zone. Smoking increases your risk for prediabetic conditions and more. Compared with nonsmoking folks who have type 2 diabetes, smokers with type 2 are three times more likely to die of cardiovascular disease.

12. Eat more often. Eating small meals frequently is better for blood sugar control than sitting down to occasional feasts. Large meals cause more glucose to enter the bloodstream quickly, taxing the ability of the pancreas to produce sufficient insulin. Studies show that people who eat smaller meals throughout the day tend to take in fewer calories and make healthier food choices.

13. Choose (a little) wine. In one study of nearly 80,000 people, women who drank beer or hard liquor one to four times a week were more likely to carry extra weight in the abdomen than women who didn't drink at all. However, wine was not associated with waist size in the study—significant because large waistlines increase diabetes risk—and might, in moderation, offer heart-protective effects that other alcoholic beverages do not.

14. Sleep for better insulin sensitivity. Recent research found that people who averaged less than 6½ hours of sleep a night were 40 percent more insulin resistant—a major risk for developing diabetes—than people who slept $7\frac{1}{2}$ hours or more. The insulin insensitivity of the short sleepers was typical of senior citizens over age 60, yet their real ages were between 23 and 42.

15. Schedule a blood sugar test. Haven't been tested? *Prevention* urges all adults to have their blood sugar checked and, if it's above normal, to take steps to lower it. A blood sugar test is an absolute must if you're 45 or older and overweight or if you have any other risk factors for diabetes. But don't stop there. You can have a serious prediabetic condition called metabolic syndrome and still have normal-looking blood sugar levels. Your answers to the next two questions will help assess your risk for this condition.

16. Look for little signs of trouble. If you have at least two of these risks—even if they seem small—plus a large waistline, odds are high that you've got metabolic syndrome. Your cells resist insulin's signal to absorb blood sugar, so your body pumps out extra blood sugar. This condition puts you at high risk for heart disease, stroke, diabetes, and other health dangers. Experts estimate that one in four, perhaps even one in two, Americans has metabolic syndrome.

17. Listen to your tape measure. Research suggests that belly fat might be an even more potent risk factor for diabetes than weight alone. While experts aren't yet sure why, one theory is that insulin resistant people store excess dietary fat in inappropriate places, such as in muscle cells and the liver, which makes it harder for their bodies to use sugar as fuel. Can't quite button your favorite jeans? Never tuck in your blouse anymore? The healthy eating tips, exercise routines, and stress-reduction tips in this book work together to help you blast belly fat. You'll look great—and feel even better.

2

The Benefits

OF BALANCE

Blood sugar control can seem complicated. But what if you had an owner's manual to your body's blood sugar control system? Here it is!

Blood sugar is not a bad guy. This sweet stuff is your body's best friend—rocket fuel for hardworking muscles and brain cells, energy that (like extra flashlight batteries or the nation's strategic oil reserves) can be stored and then released at precisely the moment you need it most.

It's only when levels rise too high—or sink too low—that blood sugar has serious, negative consequences for your mood, your weight, your energy level, your health, even your life. The trick to staying on blood sugar's good side is simple: Work with—not against—the intricate and intelligent biochemical system that keeps levels within a healthy range. Your first step? Understand how your blood sugar control system works by reading this brief owner's manual.

The Right Fuel

Nearly all the blood sugar that powers your cells comes from the carbohydrates on your plate—the fruits, vegetables, grains, and sugar that your digestive system converts into the tiniest of sugar molecules: glucose.

In a sense, carbs are like candy. Whether you're eating corn chips, chocolate mousse, or broccoli spears, carbohydrate foods all contain chains of sugar molecules. Some chains are short. Others are long. Some, such as the sugars glucose and fructose, need almost no digestion before they can be absorbed into your bloodstream. Others, like the fiber in oatmeal, are so tough that your body cannot break them down.

The moment you slide a forkful of apple pie or mashed potatoes into your mouth, a series of enzymes begins breaking apart these chains. Ultimately, all carbs are converted into glucose, fructose, or galactose, tiny sugar molecules that slide easily through your intestinal wall and into the bloodstream. There's one more stop before this new supply of blood sugar can reach hungry cells: the liver. Here, cells hold on to some glucose for later use (it's stored in a form called glycogen), and fructose and galactose are converted into glucose. Like gasoline pumped into the tank of your car at the start of a summer road trip, the glucose that circulates in your bloodstream is now ready to power your mind, muscles, and metabolism.

The Simple-Carb Myth

Until recently, nutrition experts thought that complex carbs—starches comprised of long chains of sugar molecules—were the "good" carbs that kept blood sugar low and steady. "Bad" carbs were simple sugars with short chains that were absorbed quickly. But that's old thinking. Experts now know that some simple carbs are absorbed slowly and some complex carbs convert swiftly into blood sugar.

A better ranking system: the glycemic index, which rates a food's effect on your blood sugar based on lab tests, not conjecture.

Sugar Lesson #1: Go for Low-Glycemic Carbs

Not all carbs are created equal. Some reach the finish line faster than others, and when it comes to healthy blood sugar, bet on the tortoise, not the hare.

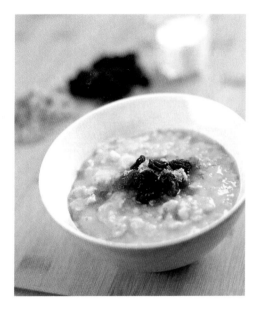

High-glycemic carbs, such as white rice and white bread, are broken down and absorbed swiftly, raising blood sugar fast. Low-glycemic carbs move through your digestive system slowly and release sugar into your bloodstream slowly. Many factors influence how rapidly or slowly a carb becomes blood sugar. Among them: whether you've also consumed something acidic (like vinaigrette dressing) or fatty (like butter on bread), both of which slow absorption; whether the starch in the food has been thoroughly cooked (the longer you cook a starch, the faster it is absorbed by your body); whether the carb is surrounded by a tough coating such as the covering on beans and seeds, which slows absorption; how finely a carb such as flour has been ground (finer grains absorb faster); and whether a carb comes with digestion-slowing viscous fiber (as do oatmeal and lentils).

Sugar Lesson #2: Burn It, or Wear It on Your Hips

Muscle cells and the tissues of organs throughout your body rely on glucose for energy to function. Walking, breathing, sweating, digesting, producing new cells, growing a baby during pregnancy, and thousands of tiny intercellular functions are all driven by this tiny sugar.

Your body's top glucose hogs are your brain and nervous system, which collectively consume about half the glucose that circulates in your bloodstream. Even at rest, the brain devours a greater percentage of your glucose supply than your body uses while active.

It takes just 7 ounces of pure glucose— less than 1 cup—to fuel the daily work and play of your cells. Like a thrifty Boy Scout, your body's glucose abides by the motto "Be prepared." About 40 percent of the glucose released after a meal is stored in the liver and muscles as glycogen. When blood sugar falls between meals or food isn't available, the liver releases its supply into the bloodstream as glucose. Muscle cells also hoard

Your Blood Sugar Timeline

The life cycle can profoundly affect blood sugar. Here's what happens.

PUBERTY

This life stage results in insulin resistance that has nothing to do with weight or fat, says Michael Goran, PhD, professor of preventive medicine at the Keck School of Medicine at the University of Southern California in Los Angeles. The cause? Probably a combination of the body's need for extra energy to fuel rapid growth and the sudden flood of sex hormones.

"Kids who go through puberty get very insulin resistant—regardless of how fat, thin, big, or small," Dr. Goran explains. If they're lean, their bodies can handle it with no long-term effects. But if they're overweight, the stress of puberty on the pancreas may push the entire system over the edge, resulting in longer-lasting insulin insensitivity or full-blown diabetes.

PREGNANCY

Nearly all pregnant women develop some insulin resistance—that is, their cells don't readily obey insulin's signal to absorb blood sugar, says Thomas A. Buchanan, MD, professor of medicine, obstetrics and gynecology, and physiology and biophysics at the Keck School of Medicine. "As you become more and more resistant to insulin, your glucose and other nutrients stay in circulation a bit longer after you eat than if your insulin reactivity were normal," explains Dr. Buchanan. "That may be a way to get some of the maternal nutrients to the fetus." In other words, more for baby.

MENSTRUATION AND MENOPAUSE

Gabriele E. Sonnenberg, MD, professor of medicine at the Medical College of Wisconsin in Milwaukee, says many of her patients with type 1 diabetes (when the immune system destroys insulin-producing cells, so you must

glycogen for their own private use. (And when your body runs out of glycogen, fat cells release fatty acids for use by skeletal muscles, your heart, and other tissues.)

Your glucose reserves must be replenished daily. Your body keeps only about 1,900 calories' worth of glycogen in its larder—enough to sustain you for about 16 hours. When that runs low, it burns fat and even uses protein to create more glucose. Most Americans have more than enough, however, thanks to overeating,

receive daily insulin injections) find it harder to control their blood sugar right before their periods. Some report problems at midcycle (during ovulation), while others say the changes come during menstruation itself. In fact, several of them change their insulin dose to coincide with their changing needs during the menstrual cycle.

Studies confirm this mysterious correlation, something women with diabetes have long experienced. In one survey of 406 women with type 1, 67 percent said they had changes in blood glucose control just before their periods and 70 percent reported changes during menstruation. Other studies find that even women without diabetes have higher blood sugar after meals during the 2 weeks between ovulation and menstruation.

Insulin may not dock as effectively with receptors on cell surfaces in the second half of the menstrual cycle, or estrogen may interact with insulin to raise or lower blood sugar.

Those cyclical/hormonal changes of menstruation should stop with menopause. But then a new factor arises: weight gain, which can increase insulin resistance and ultimately raise sugar levels.

With age, the body's ability to produce insulin and absorb blood sugar declines. Blame it on wear and tear, genetics, and a tendency to eat more and sit more. Part of the reason may lie within tiny structures inside cells, called mitochondria, the little power plants that turn glucose into energy. Mitochondria work less efficiently as we grow older, burning less blood sugar. The result: Risk for diabetes rises over age 40 and rises even faster after age 60.

The Rx: exercise. Muscle is one of the major users of glucose, Dr. Sonnenberg notes. If you maintain it with resistance training and aerobic activity, you can improve your blood sugar status at any age.

inactivity, and a taste for refined carbohydrates. When there's an overload of glucose, your liver and muscle cells can run out of storage space. The excess sugar is stored—as fat.

But if you exercise (we recommend at least 30 minutes at least five times a week), you burn more glucose, and you also activate a mechanism that pulls blood sugar into cells independent of insulin. You get a double benefit: no excess insulin, lower glucose.

Sugar Lesson #3: Protect Your Insulin Production and Insulin Sensing Systems

Normal blood sugar stays within a range of 60 to 90 milligrams of glucose per deciliter of blood (mg/dl) before a meal and rises to between 120 and 160 mg/dl after eating.

If blood sugar control is a balancing act, hormones act as the tightrope walker's pole. "Blood sugar regulation involves a balance between hormones that raise blood glucose and those that lower it," says Robert Cohen, MD, professor of medicine in the division of endocrinology and metabolism in the department of medicine at the University of Cincinnati. The key players are insulin, which lowers blood sugar by persuading cells to absorb it; and the hormone glucagon, which tells the liver to release stored glucose.

Insulin is produced by beta cells in the pancreas. Under healthy conditions, these clever cells sense glucose levels in the bloodstream and adjust their insulin output accordingly. After you eat, insulin levels rise. Once released, insulin ushers glucose out of the bloodstream and into waiting cells throughout the body. When sugar levels fall, so does insulin production.

But if you're overweight and inactive, receptors on muscle, liver, and organ cells throughout your body may grow deaf to insulin's signals. Then, your beta cells pump out extra insulin, raising your risk for stubborn overweight as well as health problems. Over time, overeating fatty and sugary foods might prompt your beta cells to lose their smart ability to sense changes in blood sugar levels. If they stop producing the right amount at the right time, blood sugar levels will rise dangerously.

Sugar Lesson #4: Take Care of Your Backup Power Supplies

If you haven't eaten in a while, alpha cells in the pancreas send glucagon into the blood. This hormone raises blood sugar by signaling the liver to give up its glycogen stores. Glycogen becomes blood sugar, ready to feed your body's fuel-hungry cells. If you overeat foods that raise blood sugar dramatically, this system can stay turned on and prevent your body from burning a secondary fuel: fatty acids stored in fat cells. This is a problem if you're trying to lose weight.

Meanwhile, chronic stress can keep another blood sugar backup plan switched on for too long. If you need a sudden burst of energy, your adrenal glands churn out stress hormones, which tell your body to release and burn stored glucose. That worked well for cavemen and cavewomen, who faced short-term stresses like marauding cats. Unfortunately, 21st-century chronic stress can keep these hormones raging, leaving you with higher blood sugar around the clock. Chronic stress can also prompt you to overeat and store extra fat in your belly, which leads to more insulin resistance. Stress reduction isn't a luxury; it's a necessity for maintaining a healthy weight!

3

Testing,

TESTING

Here's your primer for which diabetes tests to take—and how to take them correctly.

Throughout our lives, we're bombarded by numbers: the speed limit on a sign, the PIN of a bank account, the phone number of a friend. When you've been diagnosed with diabetes, suddenly some new numbers become critical—really a matter of life or death. These numbers are the measurements of your blood sugar control, and you'll learn them from certain routine diabetes tests. Your doctor will work with you to establish the best testing routine for you. Here's an idea of what to expect.

The Tests You Need

To stay healthy and avoid complications, you need tight blood sugar control. How do you know if your diet, exercise, and medication plan is really working? By testing your blood sugar every day with your blood sugar meter, and by seeing your doctor several times a year for an A1c test, which reveals your average blood sugar for the past 2 to 3 months.

"Daily checks and A1c tests look at blood sugar in two very different ways," says Francine Kaufman, MD, former president of the American Diabetes Association, former head of the Center for Endocrinology, Diabetes and Metabolism at Children's Hospital Los Angeles, and author of *Diabesity: The Obesity-Diabetes Epidemic That Threatens America—And What We Must Do to Stop It.* "A daily test is a snapshot. Taken with a blood sugar meter, it tells you what your level is at one moment. It's very useful for finding out how high your blood sugar is at key times of day—first thing in the morning before you eat, before a meal, after exercise—or to see how well your body handles the natural rise in blood sugar after you eat."

In contrast, the A1c is like a full-length movie. It tells you what's happened, on average, to your blood sugar over the past 2 to 3 months.

"With results of both tests, you can see if there's a disconnect between your diabetes management plan and your real blood sugar levels," Dr. Kaufman explains. "What if your daily checks look good, but your A1c is high? You may discover that the meter you use for daily checks isn't working right or that there's a time of day when your sugar's much higher than you ever realized. You may need to alter your medication dosage, adjust the size of your meals or your food choices, work on lowering stress, or resolve to exercise more. If you weren't getting A1c checks every few months, you'd never know there was a problem."

An A1c test measures the amount of sugar attached to hemoglobin in your bloodstream. Found inside red blood cells, hemoglobin carries oxygen from your lungs to cells throughout your body. But it also links up with sugars such as blood glucose along the way. Like Christmas cookies rolled in sweet sprinkles, hemoglobin picks up more and more sugar if there's an excess in your blood. Research confirms that every one-point rise in your A1c level significantly raises your risk for heart attack; stroke; and damage to eyes, kidneys, and nerves. An A1c above 7 percent raises heart attack risk 25 percent, ups stroke risk 30 percent, triples your chances of nerve damage in legs and feet, and raises odds for nerve damage in the eyes by up to 50 percent. Every one-point drop in your A1c cuts your risk for complications by up to 41 percent.

But daily tests are important, too. "The A1c cannot give you the quick results you need to see if a new sugar control strategy is working," Dr. Kaufman says. "You need to know right away if your medication is effective, whether a new food raises your levels too high, or how physical activity impacts your blood sugar. Everyone's body is different. Daily tests let you see just how your body is reacting, so that you can fine-tune your plan." Here's how to get the most from this testing strategy.

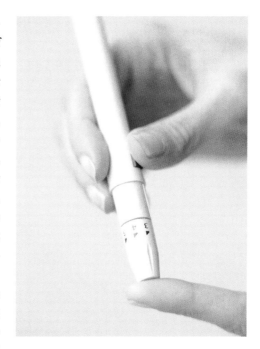

DAILY BLOOD SUGAR CHECK(S)

When to check. Work with your doctor. If you've just been diagnosed or are starting a new medication, you might need to test three to six times a day. If your treatment is working well, you might need fewer checks. If you test just once or twice a day, check at different times on different days. That will give you a more complete idea of how your sugar levels rise and fall.

Shoot for these numbers. For a fasting test (such as first thing in the morning) or before a meal, 90 to 130 mg/dl; 2 hours after a meal, less than 180 mg/dl.

Best test equipment. A glucose monitor that's less than 2 or 3 years old or an older meter that's been calibrated with your doctor's help. "After a while, meters wear out," says Karmeen Kulkarni, RD, MS, CDE, president of the ADA's health care and education program and a certified diabetes educator at St. Mark's Hospital in Salt Lake City. "New meters have some great features. You can store your previous readings, then download them into your computer, for example."

Cost. Meters may cost as little as $10 for a very basic model to more than $300 for a sleek version that doubles as a personal digital assistant (PDA). Supplies, such as lancets for drawing blood and test strips, cost extra. Check with your insurance company to see which meters they cover or how much they'll kick in. Some insurers also cover the cost of test strips.

Smart test tip. Write your results down. If you don't use a meter that automatically records your readings, keep a blood sugar log with the date, time of day, and whether it's a fasting or postmeal reading. Add comments about factors that could have influenced your reading, such as a stressful experience, a just-completed exercise routine, or a new food (or splurge). Take your records to every diabetes checkup so your doctor can review them with you.

OUCHLESS TESTING

If blood sugar checks hurt, the following strategies could help.

- Adjust your blood sugar meter so that the lancet penetrates as little skin as possible.
- Use a fresh lancet for each test. Reused lancets grow dull and hurt. (Medicare and private insurance usually cover the cost of lancets, so there's no need to save money by using them again and again.)
- Try taking your blood sample from your palm or the side of your finger instead of your finger pads. Some meters can also test on your thigh or upper arm.
- Be patient. Checking your blood sugar might soon be as easy as slicing an onion. A new study from India reveals that tears may be just as effective as blood samples at tracking blood sugar levels. The discovery will allow researchers to develop a new kind of test strip that could measure blood sugar levels simply by being placed near the corner of the eye.

A1C TEST

When to check. Every 2 to 3 months if your blood sugar is high. If it's been under tight control for a long time (at least a year), your doctor may approve twice-yearly A1c checks.

Shoot for this number. An A1c reading of 6.5 to 7. "Normal A1c levels for people without diabetes are 6 percent or lower," says diabetes specialist Jaime A. Davidson, MD, of the Dallas-based Endocrine and Diabetes Associates of Texas. "The closer to normal, the better, but be reasonable. If your A1c is high and you bring it down even somewhat, you've reduced your risk for complications."

Best test equipment. The kind at your doctor's office or a commercial lab. Home A1c tests are available for about $25, but experts recommend lab tests for more consistent results. Your doctor reads the report and can help chart your progress.

Cost. Forty dollars at a private lab. Insurance might cover most or all of the cost.

Smart test tip. Many doctors test A1c levels just once a year. Ask about more frequent checks, Dr. Davidson suggests, especially if you've started a new medicine or have difficulty keeping your daily blood sugar under control.

CHAPTER

4

Ancient Remedies,
MODERN CURES

Natural healers discovered these wonder potions hundreds
of years ago. Turns out they really were on to something.

O ver the past century, Americans have embraced modern pharmaceutical science and the lifesaving medicines it has produced. In the process, we've relegated the cures our grandparents relied on to folklore.

As it turns out, that trove is rich with effective remedies. In fact, even modern medicine relies on plants more than many of us realize, says Catherine Ulbricht, PharmD, senior attending pharmacist at Massachusetts General Hospital and chief editor of publications for the Natural Standard Research Collaboration, which evaluates scientific data on herbs.

"Practically all of the most widely used drugs have an herbal origin," Dr. Ulbricht says. "The number one OTC medication, aspirin, is a synthetic version of a compound found in the willow tree. Many statins are based on fungi; and Tamiflu originated from Chinese star anise."

Following, you'll find a host of age-old remedies whose remarkable effectiveness has been confirmed by new research. Because botanical medicines can interact with other drugs, tell your doctor when you're taking them. The exceptions are the common food items—onions, parsley, and cayenne—when consumed in natural form and conventional amounts. (To learn where to purchase herbal remedies, see "Where to Find Botanicals" at the end of this chapter.)

Onion: A Dose of Diabetes Prevention

Tradition says. Onions are considered cure-alls in many cultures. In Middle Eastern traditional medicine, they were prescribed for diabetes. During the early 20th century in the United States, William Boericke, MD, recommended onions for respiratory and digestive problems in his influential medical treatise, "Homeopathic Materia Medica." Believing that onions would help improve athletic performance, ancient Greek Olympians scarfed them down, drank their juice, and rubbed them on their bodies before competitions.

Research proves. A stack of new studies has confirmed many old-time uses of onions. Their thiosulfinates (sulfur compounds responsible for their smell) reduce diabetes symptoms and protect against cardiovascular disease. Quercetin, a flavonoid found in onions, prevents the inflammation associated with allergies and also protects against stomach ulcers and colon, esophageal, and breast cancers.

And it looks like the ancient Olympians had it right: A 2009 study in the *International Journal of Sport Nutrition and*

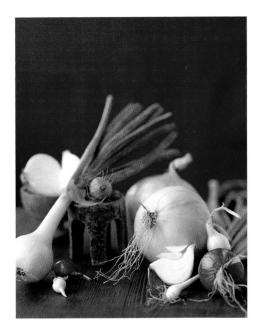

Exercise Metabolism found that quercetin extract increased endurance, making onions a perfectly legal performance-enhancing substance.

Get the benefit. Onions might keep the doctor away even better than apples do. Your body absorbs quercetin from onions at least three times faster than it does from apples (or from tea, another top source), says a report for the Federation of European Biochemical Societies. To get the most thiosulfinates, choose red or yellow onions.

"The more colorful, the better," says Michael Havey, PhD, a USDA geneticist and University of Wisconsin professor of horticulture.

Heat diminishes the thiosulfinates, so eat onions raw or lightly cooked, Dr. Havey adds. "Because of differences among types of onions and preparation methods, it's impossible to say how much to eat. Make them a regular part of a vegetable- and fruit-filled diet."

Cayenne: Blood Sugar Control

Tradition says. Columbus is credited with transporting cayenne peppers—also called chile peppers, after their Aztec name, *chil*—from the New World to the Old. Consumed in the Americas for some 7,000 years, the fiery-flavored pods reminded the explorer of black pepper, a highly prized—and pricey—spice in Europe at the time. The easy-to-grow chile pepper quickly assumed a central role in traditional cookery and remedies worldwide. Folk medicine practitioners used it for everything from pain relief to aphrodisiacs.

Research proves. Cayenne appears to control blood sugar. Study participants who ate a lunch containing capsaicin had higher blood levels of a sugar-regulating hormone and less ghrelin, the "hunger hormone," than those who ate a bland meal, reported the *European Journal of Nutrition* in 2009.

The latest research indicates that the sizzling spice might also assist in weight control. A 2009 paper in the *American Journal of Clinical Nutrition* reports that capsaicin-related compounds helped people lose abdominal fat.

Capsaicin, the ingredient that gives cayenne its heat, is best known today for pain relief—easing muscle aches, postoperative discomfort, and arthritis. Studies show that it tamps down chemical messengers that transmit pain messages in the brain.

Get the benefit. No dose has been established for blood sugar control or weight control. However, cayenne peppers are on the FDA's Generally Recognized As Safe list, so you can add fresh chile peppers to taste in your favorite dishes (or, more conveniently, powdered cayenne, available in supermarkets). Chop finely, then cook them in soups and stews or add them uncooked to salad dressings.

For pain relief, follow package instructions on OTC capsaicin ointments and creams, including Zostrix or Capzasin-HP Arthritis Pain Relief, available in drugstores or online.

Hawthorn: A Boost to the Heart

Tradition says. From China to Europe to Native America, herbalists have used hawthorn's green leaves, white or pink flowers, and tart red fall berries to strengthen cardiovascular health. "It acts on the muscle of the heart," explained Dr. Boericke in the early 20th century; he suggested prescribing it when "heart muscles seem flabby, worn out." Scientists date the use of this shrub to at least the 1st century, when Dioscorides, a famed Roman physician, wrote of it in "De Materia Medica," which became the most influential medical treatise of the next 16 centuries. In Europe and America, hawthorn jams and jellies are longtime favorites.

Research proves. Recent studies back up the old-time uses, indicating that antioxidant compounds in hawthorn relax arterial-wall muscles, increasing blood flow to the heart and preventing or reducing symptoms of coronary artery disease (CAD). Studies also show that the flavonoids may both prevent and treat additional cardiac ailments, including congestive heart failure. An analysis of existing studies done in 2008 by Cochrane Researchers found that hawthorn extract increases the heart's strength and exercise tolerance, diminishes its oxygen needs, and reduces cardiac patients' shortness of breath.

Get the benefit. If you have a cardiac condition, such as CAD, high blood pressure, or congestive heart failure, you should be under the care of a health care professional, who can advise you what form to take—tea, tincture, or capsule. Studies showing benefits for the heart used 60-milligram doses three times a day.

Lemon Balm: A Balm for the Mind

Tradition says. *Melissa officinalis,* a lemon-scented member of the mint family, has long been used to banish anxiety, boost memory, and aid sleep and digestion. It is "good against the biting of venomous beasts, comforts the heart, and driveth away all melancholy and sadnesse," wrote Elizabethan-era herbalist John Gerard in 1597.

Research proves. Stressed because of your diabetes diagnosis? Got a test, presentation, or other stress-filled occasion coming up? As in days of old, a tea made of lemon balm might help you sleep soundly the night before and keep you calm and focused at the moment of truth, says a 2003 article in *Neuropsychopharmacology.*

Research suggests this plant is effective in extreme situations, too. Four weeks of *Melissa officinalis* aromatherapy cut agitation in patients with severe dementia, reports a 2002 study in the *Journal of Clinical Psychiatry,* while 4 months of treatment with an alcohol tincture of the plant significantly reduced dementia and agitation in Alzheimer's patients, according to a 2003 article in the *Journal of Neurology, Neurosurgery & Psychiatry.*

Lemon balm appears to calm an overactive thyroid (Graves' disease), according to Eric Yarnell, ND, an assistant professor of botanical medicine at Bastyr University. It also fights viruses. Recent studies indicate that lemon balm cream speeds healing of oral herpes lesions and reduces the frequency of outbreaks.

Get the benefit. For lemon balm's calming effects, try a daily tea made with one-half to one full dropper of tincture or 1 to 2 teaspoons of dried herb steeped in 1 cup of hot water for 5 to 10 minutes, says herbalist Linda Different Cloud, a PhD candidate in ethnobotany at Montana State University. Ask your doctor first if you take thyroid medication, as

the botanical may change the amount you need.

To use *Melissa officinalis* topically, follow the instructions on OTC creams, such as Cold Sore Relief or WiseWays Herbals Lemon Balm Cream, available online or at drugstores or health food stores.

Plantain: Your Skin's Best Friend

Tradition says. Plantain, or *Plantago major,* a low-growing, oval-leafed plant found all over the globe, is a traditional remedy for skin ailments. Hildegard von Bingen, a 12th-century Benedictine abbess, healer, composer, and eventually saint, suggested applying it to insect bites in her renowned medical treatise, "Physica." Native Americans apply plantain poultices to insect stings, wounds, burns, and more, says Different Cloud, who lives on the Standing Rock Sioux Reservation in North and South Dakota. (Note: Do not confuse this leafy plant with a very different, banana-like tropical fruit that happens to have the same name.)

Research proves. The plant's antimicrobial and anti-inflammatory properties help heal breaks in the skin, researchers have found. Its soothing effects work internally, too: Psyllium, the seed of one type of plantain, is the source of the fiber in some laxatives.

Get the benefit. Plantain is difficult to identify, so you're best off buying it from an herbalist. Different Cloud recommends steeping $1/2$ cup of dried plantain in 2 cups of hot water for 10 to 15 minutes. Dip a clean cloth or compress in the warm liquid and place on skin for up to 30 minutes, changing cloths and repeating as necessary. For poison ivy, try Tecnu Rash Relief spray, which contains skin-calming plantain and the traditional itch-relieving herb *Grindelia*, available at drugstores or online.

Parsley: Urinary Tract Aid

Tradition says. Parsley root can be used for diseases of the urinary tract, wrote botanist and apothecary John Parkinson in a treatment recommendation he prepared for the queen of England in 1629. Centuries later, Dr. Boericke's "Homeopathic Materia Medica" recommended parsley for urinary tract ailments, as did *The Eclectic Materia Medica, Pharmacology and Therapeutics,* a manual of the Eclectics, a group of US physicians who practiced from the mid-1800s to the early 1900s and were famous for their use of North American botanicals.

Of course, after you've eaten all those onions as suggested earlier, you'll also need this breath freshener of yore. "The strong smell of onions is quite taken away by the eating of parsley leaves," counseled Parkinson.

Research proves. According to Yarnell's 2002 *World Journal of Urology* review of several animal studies, parsley roots do increase urine output. The German Commission E, a regulatory body, has approved the plant for cystitis and other urinary tract disorders.

Where to Find Botanicals

You can purchase the dried herbs, tinctures, and other nonfood herbal items mentioned here at Jean's Greens (518-479-0471; www.jeansgreens.com) or Starwest Botanicals (800-800-4372; www.starwest-botanicals.com). To grow herbs, find seeds at Horizon Herbs (541-846-6704; www.horizonherbs.com). And remember: When looking for a plant in the wild, bring along a field guide or other visual aid.

Get the benefit. If you have a urinary tract infection or a similar discomfort, try drinking three daily cups of tea, each made with 2 grams of common parsley (you don't need just the roots), or taking 2 to 4 milliliters of tincture three times each day for the duration of the condition.

To benefit the urinary tract long term, eat parsley leaves regularly, advises Yarnell. Munch on the sprig decorating your restaurant meal; at home, add chopped leaves to omelets, salads, and hot dishes. One more benefit of eating it: Parkinson's breath-freshening advice will work as well for you as it did for the queen of England, thanks to parsley's odor-zapping chlorophyll.

5

12 Power

HEALTH MOVES

Who says there's no such thing as instant gratification?
These minor moves offer major benefits and instant energy.

In addition to the health challenges of diabetes itself, this condition raises your risk of other health conditions as well. Everything from your heart to your mood to your weight can be affected. Here are some simple ways to ward off some diabetes complications—and some other common health problems as well.

Improve Blood Flow by 21 Percent

Laugh.

A good laugh can be good for your heart. One recent study from the University of Texas at Austin found that those who chuckled while watching a comedy increased the dilation of blood vessels by 20 percent for up to 24 hours. When they watched a serious documentary, the arteries actually constricted by 18 percent. (Constricted blood vessels can lead to high blood pressure.)

"When you're happy, your body releases feel-good neurochemicals, which can have numerous favorable effects on the body," says David Katz, MD, director of the Prevention Research Center at Yale University School of Medicine.

Cut Stroke Risk by 21 Percent

Brew a pot of tea.

Sipping tea might help protect you from a life-threatening stroke, according to a study from UCLA School of Medicine. Researchers there examined data from nine studies detailing almost 4,400 strokes among 195,000 people and found that those who drank at least three cups a day had 20 percent the risk of stroke, compared with those who drank less than one cup.

It doesn't matter if you prefer green or black tea. Both are made from the same plant, *Camellia sinensis,* whose powerful antioxidant EGCG (epigallocatechin gallate) and amino acid theanine may protect vessels and arteries.

Lose 5 Pounds

Have milk with breakfast.

Women who consumed a large (20-ounce) glass of fat-free milk in the morning ate on average 50 fewer calories at lunch, compared with days when they drank fruit juice with the same number of calories, according to a study published in the *American Journal of Clinical Nutrition.* Researchers say the milk drinkers felt more satisfied and were less likely to overeat at their next meal. Over a year, that translates to a 5-pound loss.

Lose 2 Inches from Your Belly

Ditch the remote.

When switching TV stations, put down the remote, get up, and do it manually. An

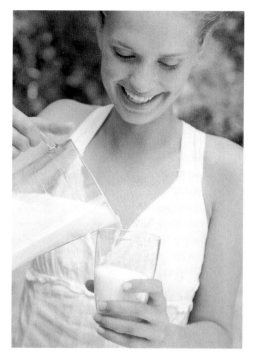

Australian study found that people who did the greatest amount of light activity during otherwise sedentary behavior, such as watching TV, had 16 percent smaller waist circumferences than those who were inclined to stay put.

Even the simple act of getting up and walking around for a minute or so was enough to make a difference, regardless of whether they had a regular workout schedule. They also had lower body mass indexes and triglyceride and glucose levels, all of which are associated with a reduced risk of metabolic syndrome. More ways to break up an otherwise inactive day: Stand up every time the phone rings at your desk; take the long way back to your desk after a bathroom break; do some stretches before reading new e-mail.

Feel 20 Percent Happier

Write a thank-you letter.

Students who wrote letters expressing gratitude to someone special were happier and more satisfied with their lives, researchers at Kent State University found. Other research has shown that expressive writing may improve immune, lung, and liver function; reduce blood pressure; and provide a greater sense of well-being. But be sincere.

"It has to be a heartfelt sentiment showing significant appreciation," says researcher Steven Toepfer, PhD, an assistant professor of family and consumer studies. Dashing off a quick e-mail or texting a pal might not have the same effect, adds Dr. Toepfer, who says taking the time to put pen to paper allowed students to reflect. "Through the process of writing, they had time to think about the links they established between themselves and others and to count their blessings a bit, which made them feel more grateful."

Cut Risk of Head and Neck Cancer by 400 Percent

Brush and floss.

Take good care of your smile, and you'll have more than just white teeth to show for it. New research from Roswell Park Cancer Institute in Buffalo, New York, shows that people with the chronic gum disease periodontitis have a fourfold risk of developing a type of head or neck cancer (which makes up about 5 percent of all malignancies in the United States), especially in the mouth and throat. The risk was increased even among patients who never used tobacco. Gum disease occurs when the bacteria that live in plaque infect the gums, so brush and floss regularly to prevent plaque buildup.

Boost Your Recall by 29 Percent

Doodle.

People who doodled while listening to a recorded message had nearly one-third better recall of the details than those who didn't draw, according to a study published in the journal *Applied Cognitive Psychology*.

"Doodling acts as a buffer against daydreaming," explains researcher Jackie Andrade, PhD, a professor in the School of Psychology at the University of Plymouth in England. "It provides just enough distraction to stop you from drifting off, but you can still focus on what is being said."

Slash Medical Mistakes by Up to 25 Percent

Follow up with your doctor.

Don't assume that no news is good news when you've had a checkup: Physicians fail to inform 1 out of every 14 patients whose abnormal test results are clinically significant, according to a recent study published in the *Archives of Internal Medicine*. Among some doctors, the number of no-calls was as high as 1 in 4. Delayed diagnoses can be linked to thousands of serious injuries and health crises—and even deaths—each year.

"If you are subjecting your vein to a needle, you have a right to know what the test is for and why it matters," says Dr. Katz. Talk with your doctor about when you'll hear about results, and if she finds something that requires treatment, when you might expect to hear from her again. You can always follow up with her after that date.

Reduce Stress by 200 Percent

Hold hands.

A brief hug and a few minutes of holding your spouse's hand can fend off stress, according to a study reported at the *American Psychosomatic Society*. Researchers asked two groups of participants to speak about a stressful event, an exercise that typically causes a spike in blood pressure. BP readings of those who did so without holding their spouse's hand before speaking were more than double those of people who held hands; their heart rates also rose twice as much.

Lower Risk of Dementia by 19 Percent

Serve fish tonight.

Here's more evidence that fish is brain food: A study of nearly 15,000 adults worldwide found that regular fish eaters (those who have it more than once a week) were just one-fifth as likely to have dementia as those who never ate the food. It also found that those whose diets contained the most meat were slightly more likely to have dementia than non-meat eaters. Omega-3 fatty acids (found in oily fish like salmon, mackerel, and tuna) might help protect nerve cells in the human brain and are known to limit inflammation, which is associated with dementia.

Ease Back Pain by 56 Percent

Do yoga.

Spending time on a yoga mat can significantly reduce chronic lower back pain, according to a study from West Virginia University. Researchers asked 45 people whose back pain caused mild to moderate disability to do a 90-minute yoga workout twice a week for 6 months. Compared with patients who only continued whatever therapy they'd already been doing, the new yogis reported significantly less pain and better function and

fewer symptoms of depression (down almost 60 percent). They also continued to see these benefits even 6 months later.

Live 5 Years Longer

Sip some merlot.

A Dutch study following 1,300 men for 40 years found that those who regularly drank up to a half glass of wine each day boosted their life expectancy by half a decade compared with teetotalers. Study authors say the polyphenolic compounds in wine (especially red) may have heart-healthy effects that are probably seen in women as well.

"Alcohol raises levels of 'good' cholesterol and can increase levels of tPA [tissue plasminogen activator], a protein that helps break down blood clots; both benefits can help minimize potentially life-threatening ailments such as stroke and heart disease," says Dr. Katz. But remember, even modest alcohol intake is associated with an increased risk of breast cancer. If you are a social drinker, keep your daily intake low—no more than one glass per day. (Men can have up to two.)

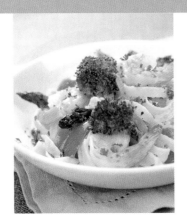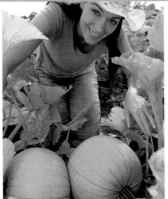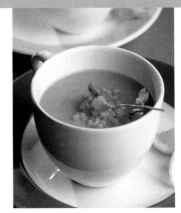

NUTRITION
Medical Breakthroughs

When you have diabetes, the phrase "you are what you eat" takes on new meaning. Here's the latest medical research on nutrition, and its impact on diabetes and blood sugar control.

START ROUGHING IT

It's no secret that fiber is essential, possibly reducing the risk of diabetes and heart disease, as well as helping us keep our appetites—and waistlines—in check. The mystery seems to be how to get enough of it. Most people consume only half of the recommended 25 to 35 grams each day. Try the following six options for something jazzier than brown rice.

Mix oats into meat loaf. Instead of nutritionally inferior bread crumbs, use ⅔ cup rolled oats per pound of meat as a binding agent. In addition to 5.5 grams of fiber, they contain magnesium, which is a mineral that might slash diabetes risk.

Make pumpkin pie oatmeal. Combine ⅓ cup canned pumpkin, 1 cup of oatmeal, 1 to 2 teaspoons brown sugar, and spices of your choice, such as cinnamon, nutmeg, or pumpkin pie spice. The pumpkin adds nearly 2.5 grams of fiber and loads of immunity-boosting vitamin A. Cinnamon in particular might be helpful for people with diabetes. Experts think this spice increases insulin action.

Spike smoothies with chocolate. A tablespoon of unsweetened cocoa powder has 2 grams of fiber, plus it contains less saturated fat than dark chocolate bars and none of the added sugars.

Toss mushrooms into soup. Rehydrate dried shiitakes in hot water for 20 to 30 minutes, then chop and add to your favorite soup for 3 grams of fiber per ounce, plus lentinan, a compound that may have anticancer properties.

Add edamame to stir-fries. Brimming with folate, a B vitamin that might protect you from pancreatic cancer, and 4 grams of fiber per ½ cup, boiled soybeans complement any Asian flavor.

Sprinkle wheat germ into pancakes. Rich in selenium, which could cut skin cancer incidence by about 60 percent, ½ cup of wheat germ packs 4 grams of fiber. Add it to any batter recipe.

TRY LENTILS

These super legumes keep blood sugar steady, which can be helpful for diabetes control. They might even cut back on hunger, boosting weight loss, according to a review of six studies.

One-quarter cup of lentils is crammed with 13 grams of protein, 11 grams of belly-filling fiber, and 5 milligrams of fatigue-fighting iron—all for only 161 calories! Harvard School of Public Health researchers found that women who ate lentils at least twice a week were 24 percent less likely to develop breast cancer than women who ate them less than once a month.

Try adding lentils to soups or salads, or mixing with whole grains. Rinse thoroughly, add to boiling water for 2 to 3 minutes, and simmer for 15 to 30 minutes before using.

Money-saving tip. Buy brown or green lentils in bulk. A pound costs about $3.

MAKE YOUR RICE NICE

If you're still eating white rice, here's yet another reason to get on the brown bandwagon. Eating brown rice just twice a week could lower your risk of type 2 diabetes 11 percent, according to a study in the *Archives of Internal Medicine*. Brown rice has more fiber, magnesium, and other nutrients shown to reduce the risk, and it causes your blood sugar to rise less rapidly after a meal than white rice does, says lead study author Qi Sun, MD, ScD.

If you don't like the taste of brown rice, try blending the two varieties until your palate becomes accustomed to it. Replacing about $1/3$ cup of cooked white with brown every day was associated with a 16 percent lower risk.

▨ GO GREEN TO STOP DIABETES

Here's great news about leafy greens: People who eat a little more than one serving (about $1^{1}/_{4}$ cups raw) daily have a 14 percent lower risk of developing type 2 diabetes, according to a recent research review. Raw or cooked, greens such as spinach, bok choy, and kale contain a triple whammy: antioxidants, which might reduce inflammation; magnesium, which has been linked to lower diabetes risk; and alpha-linolenic acid, a fatty acid that might cut insulin resistance, say researchers at the University of Leicester in England.

▨ CURB DIABETES WITH COFFEE

A deluge of new studies confirms that java delivers a major health jolt, thanks to its rich source of nutrients that improve insulin sensitivity, lower cholesterol, and destroy damaged cells. Even caffeine is protective, so don't opt for decaf unless you suffer from insomnia, headaches, or high blood pressure. Compared with people who drink the least amount of coffee, here's how your healthy habit stacks up.

At least 1 cup per day. Lowers your risk of early death from all causes by 37 percent.

At least 2 cups per day. Reduces your risk of death from heart disease by 25 percent.

At least 3 cups per day. Slashes your risk of dementia and Alzheimer's disease by 65 percent.

4 or more cups per day. Makes you 56 percent less likely to develop type 2 diabetes.

▨ EAT A RAINBOW OF HEALTH

A colorful plate delivers a hefty dose of age-fighting nutrients. The healthiest (and tastiest) diet is a colorful one, but 80 percent of Americans still don't eat enough brightly hued fruits and vegetables, according to a new analysis of the National Health and Nutrition Examination surveys. Produce contains phytonutrients, which are plant-based compounds that researchers believe might help ward off obesity, cancer, and heart disease. Here's a breakdown of what you need more of and why. Aim for two $1/_2$-cup servings from each group daily.

GREEN FRUITS AND VEGETABLES
Eat more. Lettuce, spinach, zucchini, broccoli, green beans, Brussels sprouts, and soybeans

They contain. Isothiocyanate, lutein, zeaxanthin, and isoflavones

They fight. Alzheimer's disease, macular degeneration, and lung cancer

RED FRUITS AND VEGETABLES

Eat more. Strawberries, tomatoes, apples, cranberries, watermelon, radishes, and pomegranate

They contain. Lycopene and ellagic acid

They fight. Cell damage and breast and prostate cancer

YELLOW AND ORANGE FRUITS AND VEGETABLES

Eat more. Squash, sweet potatoes, carrots, apricots, cantaloupe, oranges, corn, pineapple, and lemons

They contain. Alpha-carotene, beta-carotene, beta-cryptoxanthin, and hesperidin

They fight. Heart disease, stroke, asthma, and rheumatoid arthritis

WHITE FRUITS AND VEGETABLES

Eat more. Garlic, onions, pears, black-eyed peas, and cauliflower

They contain. Allicin and quercetin

They fight. High blood pressure, cholesterol, and bone loss

PURPLE AND BLACK FRUITS AND VEGETABLES

Eat more. Grapes, figs, blueberries, red cabbage, black currants, eggplant, black beans, and plums

They contain. Anthocyanidins and resveratrol

They fight. Memory loss, premature aging, cancer, and heart disease

◼ BE SWEET SAVVY FOR BETTER BP

People who consume more than 74 grams of added fructose a day (that's two to three sweetened soft drinks) are 87 percent more likely to have severely elevated blood pressure than those who get less, according to a recent study. Researchers believe that excess fructose might reduce the production of nitric oxide, a gas that helps blood vessels relax and dilate. Our swaps target the worst offenders (drinks and baked goods) and offer substitutions sweetened with fruit, which has less fructose and more healthy nutrients.

Swap out. Soda

Swap in. 12-ounce seltzer with frozen lemon slices

Swap out. Banana-nut muffin

Swap in. 1 whole wheat English muffin with 2 tablespoons of natural peanut butter and $\frac{1}{2}$ banana, sliced

Swap out. Oatmeal raisin cookie

Swap in. $\frac{1}{2}$ cup of oatmeal with 1 tablespoon of raisins and 1 teaspoon of cinnamon

◼ SPOT A HEALTH FOOD

Food labels don't lie. But if you're one of the 60 percent of people who rely on them to make healthy choices and you don't know what to look for, they can deceive. Kathy McManus, RD, director of the department of nutrition at Brigham and Women's Hospital in Boston, offers five ways to sleuth out the truth.

The percentage of a woman's increased odds of surviving a stroke if she has three servings of produce daily, according to the *American Journal of Clinical Nutrition.*

53

Check the servings. If one package doesn't equal one serving, multiply the nutritional information by how many you're going to eat—especially calories. Packaged meals should contain no more than 400; snacks shouldn't exceed 150.

Limit bad fats. Pick products with zero trans fat and low saturated fat. For example, women on a 1,600-calorie diet need no more than 13 grams daily.

Pick low sodium. Most people get far too much sodium, and up to 75 percent of it comes from processed foods. Full meals shouldn't exceed 500 milligrams; cap your daily intake at 2,000 milligrams.

Fill up on fiber. Foods that contain 3 grams or more can help reduce appetite and cholesterol.

Go beyond sugar grams. Some healthy foods are high in natural sugar. If the number of grams seems high, make sure the ingredient list doesn't contain added sweeteners.

■ TAKE D WITH DINNER

If you take your vitamin D supplement with the largest meal of the day, you can boost your absorption by nearly 57 percent, according to new Cleveland Clinic research. Most of us don't get enough of this powerful nutrient, which might lower diabetes risk, ward off cancer, boost immunity, prevent back pain, and more.

6

The Best Foods for People

WITH DIABETES

Fill up on these nutrients to control blood sugar and slim down.

Eating to beat diabetes is as easy as 1, 2, 3, 4. That's right, there are four fabulous food groups that will help you to control your blood sugar.

Diabetes Fighter #1: Fiber

Fill up to slim down.

Whole foods tempt us with their come-hither hues—the jewel-toned berries and lush, leafy greens; the luminous beans; the rich, earthy grains. Like bees to flowers, we're drawn to them. That's a good thing, because underneath those beautiful exteriors, whole foods pack some serious nutrition, including a mother lode of fiber.

A half century of research has proven fiber to be the Swiss Army knife of nutrients. Name just about any health problem—type 2 diabetes or high blood sugar, for example—and a high-fiber diet probably can help treat it, if not prevent it in the first place.

Trying to lose weight? Then fiber-rich foods definitely are the way to go. Case in point: Researchers at the University of Minnesota found that people who ate the most vegetables, fruits, and other fiber-rich foods lost 2 to 3 pounds more per month than those on lower-fiber diets.

With all the good things it has going for it, fiber ought to be a dietary mainstay. Yet a full two-thirds of us are getting 15 grams a day at most. That's about half of the recommended 25 to 30 grams a day!

Why are so many of us coming up so short? The answer, at least in part, is that fiber-rich whole foods must compete with processed foods for our dietary favor. The latter's very name suggests their inherent weakness: Processed foods are pretty much devoid of fiber.

THE 411 ON FIBER

So just what is fiber? Simply put, it's the component of a plant food that passes through the digestive system pretty much intact. The term *fiber* actually describes a group of plant compounds, each with different functions and health benefits and each generally categorized as soluble or insoluble.

Soluble fiber is the kind that dissolves in water and turns into a thick gel during digestion. The humble apple, which contains a modest 80 calories but an impressive 5 grams of fiber, is an excellent source of a particular soluble fiber called pectin. If the name rings a bell, it's because pectin is used as a thickener in foods like jams and jellies. The same properties allow pectin to "thicken" in your digestive tract. The result: You feel fuller after eating.

Soluble fiber's gummy texture also might interfere with carbohydrate and glucose absorption in the intestines, leading to lower blood sugar and insulin. With your blood sugar on an even keel, you're better able to manage hunger and cravings.

Another benefit of soluble fiber is its

ability to lower cholesterol. One study found that for every gram of soluble fiber consumed in a diet of primarily fruits, veggies, and whole grains, blood cholesterol could decline by as much as 2 percent.

Unlike soluble fiber, insoluble fiber—your grandmother called it roughage—doesn't dissolve in water. Because it stays solid, it adds bulk to bowel movements. It also speeds the passage of food through the digestive tract, which means the intestines have less time to absorb carbohydrates. The result: Your blood sugar stays on an even keel.

This is one reason for insoluble fiber's impressive ability to reduce diabetes risk. When Finnish researchers tracked 4,316 men and women ages 40 to 69 over 10 years, they found that the people who

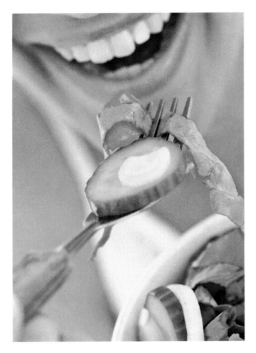

ate the most fiber from cereal grains were 61 percent less likely to develop type 2 diabetes than those who ate the least.

Among the best sources of insoluble fiber are whole wheat flour, wheat bran, and many vegetables. For soluble fiber, top-notch sources include oats, peas, beans, apples, and citrus fruits. That said, plant foods vary greatly in the types and amounts of fiber they contain. Your best bet is to vary your food choices.

FEEL FULL ON FEWER CALORIES (SERIOUSLY!)

As we mentioned earlier, fiber is a must-have for any weight-loss plan—or at least the ones that produce results. Large-scale studies have shown that people who follow high-fiber diets tend to have lower body weights and less body fat than those who don't. For example, when Tufts University researchers reviewed the findings of several weight-loss studies, they concluded that increasing fiber intake by 14 grams per day could lower a person's calorie intake by 10 percent.

Why fiber promotes weight loss isn't rocket science. First, fiber-rich foods tend to require more chewing. More chewing means it takes longer to eat a meal, which allows time for your brain to get the message that your body has gotten its fill. So, you're less likely to overeat.

Further, high-fiber foods tend to have more volume. In other words, they take up more room in your belly, so that I'm-full feeling lingers long after you've taken

EASY WAYS TO GET YOUR FIBER

We've put together a list of tips for you to follow, but don't try them all at once. Your digestive tract might not forgive you. Instead, choose one or two that seem doable to you.

- Select a breakfast cereal that provides 5 or more grams of fiber per serving. Another option: Add 2 tablespoons of unprocessed wheat bran to your favorite nonsugary cereal.

- Switch to a whole grain bread that contains at least 2 grams of fiber per serving. Read labels to make sure you're getting the real thing. You should see whole wheat, whole wheat flour, or another whole grain in the top spot on the ingredient list.

- Eat whole fruit instead of drinking fruit juice. Berries, along with pears, apples, and oranges, are good sources of fiber.

- Swap meat for legumes two or three times per week. Black beans, chickpeas, and edamame (whole soybeans) are high in fiber, low in fat, and packed with lean protein. Toss them in salads, or add them to chili or soups.

- Visit your local natural foods store and experiment with some of the more exotic whole grains, such as buckwheat, millet, barley, and quinoa.

- Take advantage of ready-to-use vegetables. Mix chopped frozen broccoli into prepared spaghetti sauce or nibble on baby carrots.

your last bite. Studies have shown that a fiber-packed breakfast—say, a slice of whole grain toast spread with peanut butter or a bowl of oatmeal with berries—reduces food intake not only for the rest of the morning, but also at lunch.

Finally, high-fiber foods deliver more food for fewer calories. A fiber-rich pear, for example, delivers 5.5 grams of fiber for a price tag of just 150 calories. Nutritionists refer to this as low energy density.

Of all the fiber-rich food choices, whole grains seem to have an especially strong connection to both weight loss and heart health. A team of researchers at the University of Pennsylvania was the first to confirm this link, in a study involving 50 overweight men and women with metabolic syndrome. All of the study participants cut their calorie intakes for 12 weeks. The key difference: Half were instructed to strive for more whole grains in their diets, while the rest were told to choose refined grains.

By the end of the study, the members of both groups had dropped between 8 and 11 pounds and showed about the same change in waistline measurements. Those eating the whole grains, however, lost a higher percentage of body fat. As a bonus, their blood levels of C-reactive protein (CRP) declined by 38 percent.

- Add some roughage to your snacks. Fresh fruits, raw vegetables with fat-free dip, and low-fat popcorn are all good choices.
- Experiment with Indian and Middle Eastern cuisines, which feature whole grains and legumes as part of the main meal. You might whip up Indian dal or Middle Eastern tabbouleh—a cracked-wheat salad flavored with lemon, fresh parsley, mint, chopped tomatoes, and spices.
- Add 1/2 cup of chickpeas, either cooked or canned, to a pot of your favorite soup. You'll boost its total fiber count by 6 grams. Be sure to rinse canned chickpeas to reduce their sodium content.
- Steam your broccoli, cauliflower, and carrots before eating them, and you'll get 3 to 5 grams of fiber per serving—up to twice the amount in the raw veggies. Heat makes fiber more available.
- Use uncooked oatmeal instead of bread crumbs in meat loaf. Add 3/4 cup of oats per pound of lean ground beef, and you'll boost the total fiber count to more than 8 grams.
- Top your fat-free ice cream with sliced fresh berries. One-half cup of raspberries provides 4 grams of fiber; the same amount of strawberries or blueberries packs 2 grams.

CRP is a marker for the chronic low-level inflammation that's a predictor of heart disease. By comparison, CRP levels remained unchanged among those eating refined grains.

Among the food sources of insoluble fiber, whole grains are the superstars. In a 2007 meta-analysis of several studies involving more than 700,000 people, researchers at the Harvard School of Public Health concluded that two extra servings of whole grains a day could reduce a person's risk of diabetes by a full 21 percent.

Across the Atlantic, German researchers made a similar finding when they tracked the eating habits of more than 25,000 men and women. Those who consumed the most fiber from whole grain cereals—about 17 grams per day—were 27 percent less likely to develop diabetes than those who ate the least (less than 7 grams per day).

AN ANSWER TO BLOOD SUGAR MEDS?

When you lose weight, you automatically improve insulin's ability to sweep blood sugar out of the bloodstream and into cells. But that isn't the only way fiber helps to rein in blood sugar. Soluble fiber appears to play an especially important role. Its secret: a quality called viscosity, which causes the stomach to empty at a more leisurely pace.

This, in turn, slows the digestion of starches and sugars and reduces spikes in blood sugar.

Among the food sources of soluble fiber are beans and legumes, which appear to work their own magic on diabetes. One noteworthy study, which appeared in the *American Journal of Clinical Nutrition,* tracked the dietary habits of 64,227 healthy middle-aged Chinese women for close to 5 years. The research team that conducted the study, from Vanderbilt University Medical Center and the Shanghai Cancer Institute in China, found that the women who consumed the most legumes were 38 percent less likely to develop type 2 diabetes. Those with high intakes of soybeans, in particular, saw their risk plummet even further—by 47 percent.

What about the fiber in fruits and veggies? Its effect on blood sugar isn't quite so clear. The German study mentioned above, for example, found no particular association between fruit and vegetable consumption and diabetes risk. On the other hand, based on data collected from more than 2,000 people over the course of 10 years, Australian researchers were able to conclude that a person could lower his or her diabetes risk by 24 percent just by eating 5 grams of fiber from vegetable sources every day.

So eat your fruits and veggies—and your beans and whole grains. No matter where you're getting your fiber, it's going to do your blood sugar a whole lot of good. Actually, fiber works so well that if you take insulin or diabetes medication, you might need to lower your dosage (with your doctor's okay, of course).

Diabetes Fighters #2 and #3: Calcium and Vitamin D

They're the dynamic duo of diabetes control.

Surprised to see calcium and vitamin D among our diabetes fighting 4? We admit, they probably are not the first nutrients that come to mind for weight loss or diabetes management. Strong bones and teeth? Definitely. Healthy blood pressure and cholesterol? Perhaps.

But the latest evidence from the research front is impossible to ignore: The combination of calcium and vitamin D appears to enhance fat burning as well as cellular insulin response. That's a surefire formula for better blood sugar control!

Despite their impressive and growing resumés of health benefits, both calcium and vitamin D tend to come up short in the typical American diet. When you think about it, this could help explain—to some degree—why obesity and diabetes have become so prevalent here.

We often recommend a D supplement of up to 800 to 1,000 IU daily—less if you live in a year-round warm climate. You might benefit from supplemental calcium, too, depending on your age and health status. As much as possible, though, we want you to get your calcium and vitamin D from foods. The reason:

There may be nutritional "supporting players" in foods that allow the superstars to work their magic. Oh yes, and foods are so much more satisfying and delicious than supplements!

CALCIUM PUTS FAT CELLS ON A DIET

Around the time you were learning about the basic four food groups in elementary school, you probably got a lesson or two about how milk—and, more precisely, the calcium in milk—helps build your bones. In fact, about 99 percent of the calcium in your body resides in your bones and teeth. The remaining 1 percent has a lot going on, too—helping your heart to beat, your blood to clot, and your nerves to communicate with each other. As you can see, your body needs calcium to thrive.

It's only fairly recently that researchers began to suspect a connection between calcium and weight loss. In 2002, a research team at the University of Tennessee put 32 people—all overweight—on calorie-restricted diets that included varying amounts of dietary calcium. Over the 6 months of the study, the people who ate three servings of dairy (including low-fat milk, cheese, and yogurt) lost 70 percent more weight—an average of 24 pounds—and 64 percent more body fat than those who ate just one serving a day.

Understandably, this study made national headlines. Ever since, experts have been debating the role of calcium—mainly from dairy foods—in weight loss.

Now, common sense will tell you that you can't expect to slim down by eating a pint of Ben & Jerry's every day. (We know. We're disappointed, too!) On the other hand, if you make a point of stocking your daily diet with low-fat, calcium-rich choices, you will stack the weight-loss odds in your favor.

So how might calcium help burn body fat? Researchers are still looking for the answer. One theory, from Michael Zemel, PhD, who led the University of Tennessee study, focuses on the role of the hormone calcitriol in fat cells.

Here's how it might work: Low blood levels of calcium cause levels of calcitriol to rise. In response, the body hoards calcium by sending more into fat cells, prompting the cells to store more fat and burn less. The reverse also appears to be true: In a calcium-rich diet, calcitriol production falls, and less calcium is shuttled into fat cells. So less fat is stored and more is burned. In essence, a lack of calcium somehow makes fat cells hang on to fat—perhaps an evolutionary vestige of our caveman ancestors, whose bodies adapted to endure times of famine.

The University of Tennessee study relied on dairy foods to cover the participants' calcium needs. At least for weight loss, foods seem a better choice than calcium supplements. It's the total mix of nutrients in foods that provides the benefit, rather than calcium in isolation.

Considering all the fabulous foods that

double as outstanding calcium sources, it's hard to fathom that we're not getting enough of the mineral in our daily diets. Yet many of us are missing the mark. According to a 2008 study, only 40 percent of American women between ages 20 and 49 are at or above the recommended intake of 1,000 milligrams of calcium a day; among women over 50, just 27 percent are getting the recommended 1,500 milligrams a day. (Calcium levels are of particular concern for women, because they're much more likely than men to develop osteoporosis.)

From D-Ficiency to D-Fense

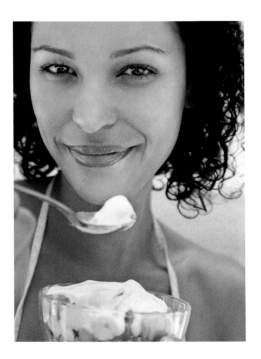

We can't really talk about calcium without bringing vitamin D into the conversation, because vitamin D's most important function is to help the intestines absorb calcium. At the risk of stating the obvious, if your gut can't absorb calcium, your body can't use it.

As you'll see a bit later in the chapter, calcium and vitamin D appear to work together to help fight type 2 diabetes. But vitamin D has benefits in its own right: It has shown promise in helping to protect against heart disease, as well as certain cancers and autoimmune diseases.

Just as with calcium, many of us—an estimated 60 percent of Americans—aren't getting enough vitamin D, according to a survey by the Centers for Disease Control and Prevention. If we're low on vitamin D, then our shortfall of calcium

makes sense. As we said earlier, our bodies can't use calcium without vitamin D. People who are deficient in vitamin D typically absorb just 10 to 15 percent of their dietary calcium, compared with 30 to 40 percent for people who are meeting their vitamin D needs.

If you're over age 50 or African American, or if you're vegan or lactose intolerant, you're more likely to experience a vitamin D deficiency than the general population. Overweight may be a risk factor, too. Though the body stores vitamin D in fat and releases it into the bloodstream on an as-needed basis, this process doesn't go quite so smoothly in the presence of extra pounds. Instead, excess body fat seems to act as a sort of trap, preventing vitamin D from entering the bloodstream.

One other possible explanation for our national vitamin D deficit: sunscreen. The human body synthesizes its own vitamin D when exposed to the sun's ultraviolet rays. Though it's highly controversial, a growing number of experts believe that since we've become so indoctrinated in the use of sunscreen, we don't give sunlight a chance to penetrate our well-protected hides. In effect, we're setting ourselves up for deficiency.

Our bodies need all the vitamin D they can get, whether it comes from sunlight (about 10 minutes a day of unprotected exposure), from food, or from supplements—or, ideally, a combination of the three.

The Antidiabetes "A Team"

If calcium and vitamin D can do so much good individually, just imagine their potential when they work together! This powerhouse pair may turn out to be the most potent diabetes defense around.

When researchers at the Tufts-New England Medical Center (now Tufts Medical Center) and other Boston-area institutions launched their exploration of the relationship between calcium and vitamin D, and type 2 diabetes, they already knew that other research findings had linked low blood levels of vitamin D to insulin resistance and type 2 diabetes. Their landmark study, published in 2006, provided compelling evidence that adequate amounts of vitamin D, in tandem with calcium, reduce diabetes risk.

For their analysis, the research team collected data from 83,779 women who already had enrolled in the long-running Nurses' Health Study. Every 2 to 4 years over the course of 2 decades, the researchers assessed the women's intakes of calcium and vitamin D from both foods and supplements.

At the outset, none of the women was diabetic. That changed by the study's end, when more than 4,800 women had been diagnosed with the disease. But the researchers also noticed this: The women who had been taking in more than 1,200 milligrams of calcium and more than 800 IU of vitamin D a day were 33 percent less likely to have developed diabetes than women who had been getting lesser amounts of both nutrients.

A more recent study, also from Tufts, determined that chronically low levels of vitamin D could raise a person's risk of type 2 diabetes by as much as 46 percent. In this meta-analysis, people who were consuming between three and five servings of dairy foods a day—including milk, which typically is fortified with vitamin D—were 14 percent less likely to develop diabetes than those who were taking in less than $1^1/_2$ servings a day.

Interestingly, this research team did not believe that getting more vitamin D by itself would be enough to stop diabetes. Drawing on other published evidence, they

EASY WAYS TO GET YOUR CALCIUM AND VITAMIN D

When you consider all that calcium and vitamin D can do for your body, you have plenty of good reasons to make sure you're getting enough of both nutrients.

Dairy is just about the best dietary source of calcium around. Just three glasses of fortified fat-free milk offer more than 1,000 milligrams of calcium, plus 400 IU of vitamin D. But what if you can't do dairy because you're lactose intolerant? One option is to use lactose-free or soy-based products; the fortified varieties are just as nutritious as the real thing, and they taste great, too! You also might try using Lactaid or another supplement that contains lactase, an enzyme that helps your body digest lactose. You can get significant amounts of calcium from nondairy sources like fortified tofu; canned salmon and sardines (with their bones); and dark green, leafy vegetables.

As for vitamin D, if the latest research is any indication, even current government guidelines—which range from 200 IU to 600 IU, based on age—may be falling short. How much higher they ought to be is the subject of considerable debate. Based on what we know so far, we think it makes good sense for everyone to take supplemental vitamin D.

Plus, on a sunny (or even cloudy) day, as you take your dog for a stroll or just walk to the mailbox and back, the sun's ultraviolet B rays strike your skin, literally creating vitamin D.

---

concluded that the combination of calcium and vitamin D—in daily doses of 1,200 milligrams and 1,000 IU, respectively—would be the most effective preventive.

Because the Tufts studies were population-based, they don't reveal precisely how calcium and vitamin D might help to derail diabetes. One explanation is that the two nutrients might enhance cellular insulin response and reduce chronic inflammation, which is a known diabetes risk factor.

The calcium–vitamin D combination is a boon to weight loss, too—though in at least one way that you might not expect. According to a 2008 study published in the *Journal of Nutrition,* this talented team helps protect against the weakening of bones that sometimes occurs in dieters. For this study, researchers at the University of Illinois assigned 130 middle-aged, overweight men and women to one of two groups. One group followed a diet that provided three servings of dairy products a day and derived 30 percent of total calories from protein, 40 percent from carbs, and 30 percent from fat. The diet for the other group had a slightly different mix of macronutrients—15 percent of calories from protein, 55 percent from carbs, and 30 percent from fat—and just two servings of dairy a day.

Over the course of 12 months, the researchers tracked the weight, bone mineral content, and bone density of all

How much vitamin D your skin makes depends on several factors, including where you live, what season and time of day it is, whether there's cloud cover or smog, and whether you're wearing sunscreen.

Age and skin color play roles, too. People over 50 don't synthesize vitamin D as well as younger folks. In fact, an average 70-year-old makes only 25 percent as much vitamin D as a 20-year-old. Melanin, the pigment that gives skin its color, also affects its ability to produce vitamin D; generally, the higher the concentration of melanin, the lower the level of vitamin D. That's why black Americans have half as much vitamin D in their blood, on average, as whites.

Given all the warnings about excessive sun exposure causing wrinkles and skin cancer, you may be concerned about soaking up the sun's rays. No worries! All you need is 10 to 15 minutes of sun time to synthesize a healthy dose of vitamin D safely.

Simply head outside on a sunny day, leaving your arms and legs uncovered. (But do protect your face, which has thinner, more sensitive skin.) Forgo the sunscreen for this brief period of time, because it hinders your body's ability to make vitamin D. After 15 minutes, you should apply sunscreen if you're planning to stay outdoors. Use a product with an SPF of at least 15, even on hazy or cloudy days.

the participants. The results: Bone density remained stable in the first group but declined in the second group. The researchers concluded that the combination and/or interaction of calcium and vitamin D with dietary protein helped to protect the participants' bones while they slimmed down.

Diabetes Fighter #4: Omega-3s

They're good for your heart—and your waistline.

If fat were a celebrity, all of Hollywood would be lining up to hire its publicist. Talk about an image transformation! A mere decade or so ago, America had become a no-fat zone, with dietary fat being blamed for health concerns from weight gain to heart disease. But something odd happened: Even though we were cutting our fat intake, we weren't getting any healthier, and our waistlines weren't getting any narrower.

It seems that in our zeal to slash fat, we were depriving our bodies of an important macronutrient. That's right: Our bodies depend on fat to function as they should. Maybe we had been consuming too much of it, but then we drifted to the other extreme, consuming way too little. As it turns out, we have to eat fat to lose weight!

Most experts agree that the right fats, in the right amounts, can be—make that should be—part of a healthy diet. By the right fats we mean omega-3 fatty acids, the kind that help melt away pounds and lower heart disease risk (which tends to be higher in those with blood sugar issues). These fats also might improve cells' insulin response!

You can get omega-3s from a variety of foods, including fish, walnuts, and flaxseed. Of these, cold-water fish, such as salmon, albacore tuna, and sardines, are by far the most abundant sources of the two types of omega-3s: eicosapentaenoic acid (EPA) and docosahexaenoic acid (DHA). (Don't worry; you're only eating them, not pronouncing them!)

GOOD FATS MAKE A COMEBACK

Fish—and therefore omega-3s—have been a staple of the human diet since, well, our caveman ancestors mastered the skill of catching them. From an evolutionary perspective, our bodies are hardwired to require these beneficial fats to carry out their most basic biochemical tasks.

Still, omega-3s are relative newcomers to the nutritional scene. In fact, they were on the verge of extinction from our modern diet, with agricultural practices and cooking methods nearly eliminating them from our food supply.

Today, omega-3s seem to be just about everywhere. Just push your cart through the aisles of any supermarket and you'll find omega-3s added to all manner of foods and beverages, including breakfast cereals, eggs, orange juice, and margarine. Even some pet foods have them! It shows how far these beneficial fats have come, capturing the attention of nutrition scientists and food manufacturers alike.

The potential health benefits of omega-3s first came to light in the mid-1970s, when a Danish research team conducted observational studies of Greenland Inuits. This population showed a very low rate of heart disease, which the researchers attributed to their traditional diet rich in fish. Since then, other observational studies have drawn a similar conclusion: Populations that eat fish on a regular basis, such as native Alaskans and Japanese, have low rates of death from heart disease. Omega-3s appear to protect the heart by reducing inflammation, preventing the blood clots that can cause heart attacks, slowing a rapid heartbeat, and relaxing the blood vessels so blood can flow freely.

Omega-3s are fats of the unsaturated variety—a category that also includes nut oils and vegetable oils. Omega-6s, found in vegetable oils as well as breakfast cereals and whole grain breads, come under the unsaturated umbrella as well. Though our bodies need both kinds of omegas, we tend to eat them in disproportionate amounts—roughly 15 to 17 times more omega-6s than omega-3s. The ratio of the two should be just about equal. When it isn't, and it stays out of sync for a prolonged period, it can pave the way for an assortment of health problems, including heart arrhythmias, depression, and certain autoimmune and inflammatory diseases.

Banisher of Body Fat, Slayer of Fat Cells

When you're getting enough omega-3s in your diet, they can do some pretty amazing things for you. Some of the most exciting research currently under way is exploring the potential for omega-3s to help shrink your waistline.

Like all other fats—whether good or bad—omega-3s promote satiety, the feeling of contentment at the end of a meal that signals you've eaten your fill. (That's why most of us would scale a 10-foot fence if we knew a full-fat chocolate chip cookie was waiting on the other side.)

Omega-3s may go one better, however. The results of a 2007 study published in the *American Journal of Clinical Nutrition* suggest that omega-3s may help burn body fat, shrink abdominal fat cells, and thwart certain genes that trigger inflammation in belly fat.

For this study, a team of French researchers assigned 27 women with type 2 diabetes to one of two groups. All the women consumed a diet that provided 55 percent of calories as carbohydrates, 15 percent as protein, and 30 percent as fat. In addition, one group took 3,000 milligrams of omega-3s in supplement form every day, while the other group got a placebo.

Over the next 2 months, the researchers tracked the women's blood sugar and insulin sensitivity, as well as their body weight, body mass index, and body fat percentage. The researchers also measured blood levels of certain substances that cause inflammation. (It's known that carrying excess body fat raises blood levels of these substances, while losing weight reduces their numbers and also improves insulin sensitivity.)

By the end of the study, women who took the omega-3 supplement had lost significantly more trunk fat—3 pounds of it, compared with less than $1/2$ pound for those taking the placebo—yet their body weights remained the same. Moreover, their fat cells shrank by 6.2 percent, while the fat cells in the placebo group actually got bigger (by only 1.2 percent, but still!). Other markers, such as blood sugar and insulin sensitivity, remained about the same for both groups.

Another study, this one conducted by researchers at the University of Georgia in Athens, investigated the effect of DHA—which, you'll remember, is a specific type of omega-3—on immature fat cells. The researchers harvested these cells, called preadipocytes, from laboratory mice. They discovered that DHA—in amounts that we humans can get from foods and supplements—may prevent the formation of new fat cells and encourage existing fat cells to kill themselves (a process known as programmed cell death, or apoptosis).

In this study, DHA appeared to encourage fat cells to release their stores of fatty acids, which is what we mean when we talk about burning fat. The researchers concluded that if people consume more omega-3s, their reward might well be flatter bellies and a lower risk of overweight and metabolic syndrome.

EASY WAYS TO EAT MORE OMEGA-3S

Here are some ways to take advantage of these beneficial fats.

- Rebalance your dietary ratio of omega-3s to omega-6s. It's simple: As you increase your intake of omega-3-rich foods, cut way back on processed foods, refined grains, and supermarket cooking oils—the chief sources of omega-6s in the average diet.
- Munch this salad every day—a potent combo of leafy greens and veggies dressed with walnut, canola, or flaxseed oil and a sprinkling of sesame seeds.
- Eat salmon or another type of cold-water fish two or three times a week. You'll get those beneficial omega-3s—and if the fish is replacing red meat in your diet, you'll probably be consuming less saturated fat.
- For lunch, help yourself to a tuna sandwich. Make your tuna with canola oil mayo.
- Try tofu—really! Tofu and other products made with soybeans are good sources of omega-3s. You can always add tofu to stir-fries, but for variety, try pureeing it with peanut butter for a fluffy sandwich spread or blending soft tofu with a banana for a breakfast smoothie.
- Add 1½ tablespoons of ground flaxseed or 1 teaspoon of flaxseed oil to your diet every day. You can mix the seeds into low-fat cottage cheese or the oil into a smoothie.
- Use canola oil to cook and flaxseed oil for salad dressings. (Flaxseed oil breaks down when it's heated, so it's not good for cooking.)
- Eat walnuts. As nuts go, they're the only kind rich in omega-3s. They may be good for the heart, too. When researchers in Spain asked a group of volunteers to eat 8 to 13 walnuts a day in tandem with a heart-healthy diet, this group showed 64 percent stronger artery-pumping action and 20 percent fewer of the gunky molecules that lead to atherosclerotic plaque than did a control group who followed the heart-healthy diet but skipped the nuts.

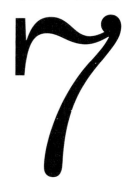

CHAPTER

Is Your Produce Losing HEALTH POWER?

Yes. Our fruits and veggies are not as nutritious as they used to be, but there's plenty you can do about it.

While we've been dutifully eating our fruits and vegetables all these years, a strange thing has been happening to our produce. It's losing its nutrients. That's right: Today's conventionally grown produce isn't as healthful as it was 30 years ago, and it's only getting worse. The decline in fruits and vegetables was first reported more than 10 years ago by English researcher Anne-Marie Mayer, PhD, who looked at the dwindling mineral concentrations of 20 UK-based crops from the 1930s to the 1980s.

It's happening to crops in the United States, too. In 2004, Donald Davis, PhD, a former researcher with the Biochemical Institute at the University of Texas at Austin, led a team that analyzed 43 fruits and vegetables from 1950 to 1999 and reported reductions in vitamins, minerals, and protein. Using United States Department of Agriculture data, he found that broccoli, for example, had 130 milligrams of calcium in 1950. Today, that number is only 48 milligrams. What's going on?

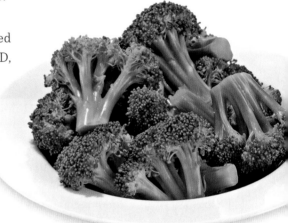

CALCIUM: **In 1950: 130 mg. Today: 48 mg**

Dr. Davis believes it's caused by the farming industry's desire to grow bigger vegetables faster. The very things that speed growth—selective breeding and synthetic fertilizers—decrease produce's ability to synthesize nutrients or absorb them from the soil.

A different story is playing out with organic produce. "By avoiding synthetic fertilizers, organic farmers put more stress on plants, and when plants

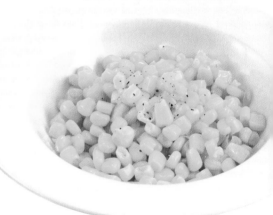

VITAMIN A: **In 1950: 390 IU. Today: 281 IU**

A Cheapskate's Guide to Organic

Smart shoppers buy organic. Smarter shoppers find ways to buy organic for less. Here's how.

Shop online. Visit www.localharvest.org to find an organic farm (or farmers' market) in your area. Many allow you to pick your own produce. Prices at local farms tend to be lower because you're essentially shopping wholesale.

Buy in bulk. In general, buying in bulk is more economical at a farm (or farmers' market) than in supermarkets.

Compare prices. Private-label organic food lines, such as Whole Foods' 365 Organic Everyday Value, can be as much as 20 percent cheaper than brand-name organic foods.

Join a food co-op. These member-owned businesses provide discounted groceries—and fresh, often organic, produce.

Freeze unused produce. Most fruits and veggies (except for whole potatoes) can be frozen for future use.

experience stress, they protect themselves by producing phytochemicals," explains Alyson Mitchell, PhD, a professor of nutrition science at the University of California, Davis. Her 10-year study in the *Journal of Agricultural and Food Chemistry* showed that organic tomatoes can have as much as 30 percent more phytochemicals than conventional ones.

But even if organic is not in your budget, you can buck the trend. We polled the experts and found nine simple ways to put the nutrient punch back in your produce.

Sleuth out strong colors. "Look for bold or brightly hued produce," says Sherry Tanumihardjo, PhD, an associate professor of nutritional sciences at the University of Wisconsin-Madison. A richly colored skin (think red leaf versus iceberg lettuce) indicates a higher count of healthy phytochemicals. Dr. Tanumihardjo recently published a study showing that darker orange carrots contain more beta-carotene.

Pair your produce. "When eaten together, some produce contains compounds that can affect how we absorb their nutrients," explains Steven Schwartz, PhD, a professor of food science at Ohio State University. His 2004 study of tomato-based salsa and avocado found this food pairing significantly upped the body's absorption of the tomato's cancer-fighting lycopene. Go to prevention.com/healthypowerpairs for more examples.

Buy smaller items. Bigger isn't better, so skip the huge tomatoes and giant peppers. "Plants have a finite amount of nutrients they can pass on to their fruit, so if the produce is smaller, then its level of nutrients will be more concentrated," says Dr. Davis.

Pay attention to cooking methods. Certain vegetables release more nutrients when cooked. Broccoli and carrots, for example, are more nutritious when steamed than when raw or boiled. The gentle heat softens cell walls, making nutrients more accessible. Tomatoes release more lycopene when lightly sautéed or roasted, says

Johnny Bowden, PhD, nutritionist and author of *The Healthiest Meals on Earth.*

Eat within a week. "The nutrients in most fruits and vegetables start to diminish as soon as they're picked, so for optimal nutrition, eat all produce within one week of buying," says Preston Andrews, PhD, a plant researcher and associate professor of horticulture at Washington State University. "If you can, plan your meals in advance and buy only fresh ingredients you can use that week."

Keep produce whole. Precut produce and bagged salads are time-savers. But peeling and chopping carrots, for example, can sap nutrients. Plus, tossing peels deprives you of good-for-you compounds. If possible, prep produce just before eating, says Dr. Bowden. "When sliced and peeled or shredded, then

The reduction in calories eaten all day after an egg and toast breakfast, according to *Nutrition Research.*

CRACK OPEN A STRONGER BODY

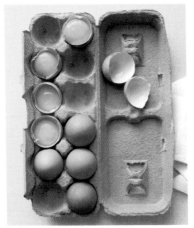

Power up omelets and frittatas by eating your eggs fresh off the farm. Researchers at Pennsylvania State University found that pasture-raised hens produce eggs with higher levels of essential nutrients than caged hens do. Pastured eggs have double the vitamin E, which strengthens your immune system, and $2\frac{1}{2}$ times as much omega-3 fatty acids, which are the nutritional heroes that aid your vision, brain functioning, and heart. To find a farm or farmers' market that sells pastured eggs, go to www.eatwild.com.

The Organic Calorie Conundrum

When you want a treat, don't judge a cookie by its label. According to a recent study, people believe that organic cookies contain 40 percent fewer calories than regular, which is a myth that can lead to overeating.

The term "organic" creates a health halo, says Jenny Lee of the Cornell University Food and Brand Lab. While the glow may be deserved for fruits and vegetables (several studies show organic versions contain more nutrients than conventionally grown), not so for packaged foods. "Organic" cookies might contain ingredients grown without conventional pesticides, but in some cases they have more calories. Treat organic cookies like any other dessert—enjoy them in moderation.

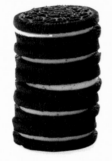

Newman's Own Organics Newman-O's

325 calories in five cookies

Oreo Sandwich Cookies

267 calories in five cookies

shipped to stores, their nutrients are significantly reduced."

Look for new colors. If you're used to munching on red tomatoes, try orange or yellow, or serve purple cauliflower along with your usual white. "Many of us buy the same kinds of fruits and vegetables each week," says Dr. Andrews. "But there are hundreds of varieties besides your usual mainstays, and their nutrient levels can differ dramatically. In general, the more varied your diet is, the more vitamins and minerals you'll get."

Opt for old-timers. Seek out heirloom varieties like Brandywine tomatoes, Early Jersey Wakefield cabbage, Golden Bantam corn, or Jenny Lind melon. Plants that were bred prior to World War II are naturally hardier because they were established—and thrived—before the development of modern fertilizers and pesticides.

Find a farmers' market. Unlike prematurely picked supermarket produce, which typically travels hundreds of miles before landing on store shelves, a

ARE YOU SHORT ON C?

Has vitamin C disappeared from your diet? Recent research found that 47 percent of people had too-low levels, even though just a 4-ounce glass of orange juice delivers nearly the daily amount you need.

People with the lowest levels of vitamin C were likelier to have a higher BMI (body mass index), waist circumference, and blood pressure than people with adequate vitamin C. The vitamin protects against inflammation, and your body uses it to build fat-burning compounds.

Not an OJ fan? Other excellent sources include red bell peppers, broccoli, cauliflower, and even romaine. Many multivitamins contain the recommended daily intake, so you don't need a separate vitamin C supplement.

farmers' market or pick-your-own venue offers local, freshly harvested, in-season fare that's had a chance to ripen naturally, which is a process that amplifies its amount of phytonutrients, says Dr. Andrews. "As a crop gets closer to full ripeness, it converts its phytonutrients to the most readily absorbable forms, so you'll get a higher concentration of healthful compounds."

8

The Dirty

DOZEN

Eating healthy foods, such as fruits and vegetables, is critical for people with diabetes. Yet it takes a toxic soup of chemicals and pesticides to get certain produce to your local supermarket. Here are the worst offenders and tips to lower your risk of exposure.

S can any supermarket produce section and what do you see? Rows of brightly hued, blemish-free fruits and vegetables. They're gorgeous. But stop and ask yourself: Without help, could nature consistently deliver such picture-perfect greens and berries, any more than it fashions every woman into a beauty pageant contestant? Of course not. Plants, like people, have natural imperfections, and some require more help than others to look good, not to mention to maintain their youthful looks as they age.

In the plant world, the equivalent of beauty products are the dozens of chemicals that farmers use to fend off insects, pests, weeds, fungal attacks, and rot. Not surprisingly, plants that are more vulnerable to attack need more of them. To help you tell which is which (and, therefore, which are best to eat organic, as opposed to those you can buy conventionally to save money), the Environmental Working Group publishes two lists—the Dirty Dozen and the Clean 15. The EWG rankings are based on USDA-tested levels of chemical residues that remain on conventionally raised fruits and vegetables after washing. Revised lists came out in 2010, with a couple of surprising new additions.

But if you should find yourself in the grocery store without the lists in hand, not to worry. There are logical reasons some types of produce are "dirtier" than others. The clues are in the plants. Read their stories, and you'll never wonder again which is which—and where you can economize.

Buy Organic—It's Worth It

Celery. Because of peak consumer demand around Thanksgiving and Christmas, 75 percent of the crop is grown during the fall and winter, when rain and wind promote the growth of bacteria and fungal diseases. Because we eat the entire stalk, it must be sprayed repeatedly to ward off pests.

"Nobody likes to find a caterpillar-damaged stalk in their celery bunch," says Stuart Reitz, PhD, a research entomologist with the USDA.

Peaches. Sweet and succulent, peaches can be just as alluring to insects as to people. Farmers might spray peaches every week or two from bloom to harvest, and peach fuzz can trap pesticides, says peach breeder John R. Clark, PhD, a horticulturalist at the University of Arkansas, who peels every one of the thousands of peaches he eats each year.

Strawberries. Strawberries are sweet and juicy, and they're also delicate and prone to disease, including fungal attacks that can turn them to mush during transit and storage.

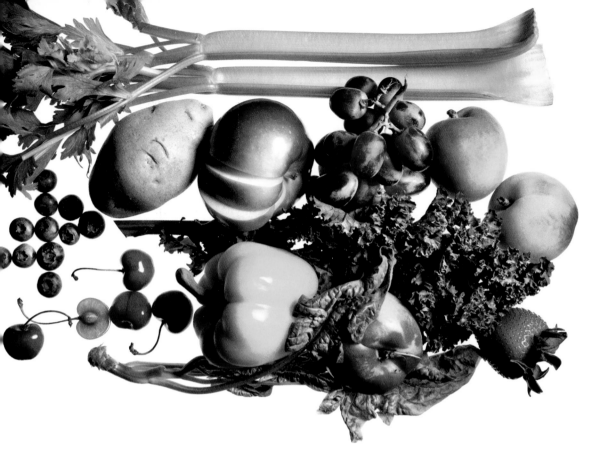

"With apples and peaches, a lot of spray-ing is cosmetic to get blemish-free fruits," says Richard Wiles, senior vice president for policy at EWG. "With berries, you're just trying to get them across the finish line into the store before they go bad."

Apples. Sweet-smelling and delicious, apples are susceptible to more than 30 insects and at least 10 diseases. Fun-gicides and other chemicals are added after picking to prevent tiny blemishes that can accumulate during storage of up to 9 months.

Blueberries. Blueberries are new on the Dirty Dozen list—possibly because the USDA began testing them only 3 years ago, after large increases in production.

The Dirty Dozen

Go Organic

Celery

Peaches

Strawberries

Apples

Blueberries

Nectarines

Bell peppers

Spinach

Kale

Cherries

Potatoes

Imported grapes

The berries are targets for insects such as blueberry maggots and bagworms.

Nectarines. Nectarines differ from peaches only in the absence of fuzz—a trait that likely arose as a natural mutation of a peach tree—so it's no wonder they're susceptible to many of the same pests, including oriental fruit moths and peach twig borers. Thanks to their waxy skin, they don't retain as many pesticides as peaches. On the other hand, they are more vulnerable to rot and scarring.

Bell peppers. Unlike cruciferous vegetables such as broccoli, sweet bell peppers (which are technically fruits) have no bitter compounds to serve as built-in insect repellents. They even lack the fiery taste of their cousins, the chile peppers. The creases at their crowns may provide nooks for pesticides to accumulate, says Philip Stansly, PhD, an entomologist at the University of Florida.

Spinach. Spinach is a mere leaf that's crunched by a variety of insects, including grasshoppers. In addition, says Wiles, "spinach tends to pull persistent DDT residues out of the soil and into the leaf." These chemicals remain in the earth decades after they were banned.

Kale. The outer leaves are not removed before sale, so any amount of damage will make kale unmarketable. Even natural enemies of the pests that feed on kale can be considered contaminants in harvested produce, so farmers spray for all bugs, including the "good" ones.

Cherries. Because cherries are a naked fruit—without peel or protection—they're vulnerable to pests such as the western cherry fruit fly. If just one of its maggots is found in a shipment, the entire load of fruit must be dumped, according to quarantine regulations, so growers spray out of fear of losing their crops.

Potatoes. New to the list, America's number one vegetable is sprayed five or more times throughout the growing season to protect against various pests—and to ensure a crop of uniform shape and size for fast-food outlets and potato chip producers. After harvesting, another round of spraying occurs in the packing shed to ward off molds and sprouting.

Imported grapes. During their long transit from the Southern Hemisphere, imported grapes are susceptible to *Botrytis cinerea* rot, which causes the fruits to split and leak. To prevent that, farmers spray aggressively with fungicides. (Domestic table grapes do not need the same spraying because most are grown in the dry desert climate of Southern California, where botrytis does not thrive.)

Buy Regular—And Save Money

Onions. Onions manufacture their own protective chemicals, a series of unpleasant-tasting sulfur compounds that discourage insect munching. Though farmers may spray early in the growing season, residues are removed when the dry outer layer of the bulb is shed during harvest.

The Clean 15

Pick Regular

Onions
Avocado
Sweet corn
Pineapple
Mangoes
Sweet peas
Asparagus
Kiwifruit
Cabbage
Eggplant
Cantaloupe
Watermelon
Grapefruit
Sweet potato
Honeydew melon

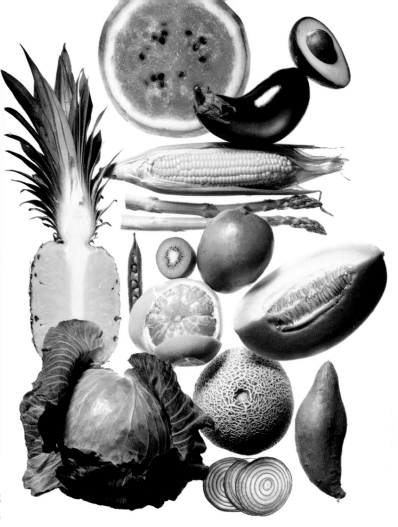

Avocado. Most of the pesticides that are used to treat avocados accumulate on the peel.

Sweet corn. Corn is husked before eating, eliminating residues on the outside.

Pineapple. Most spraying is done early in the growing season, so minimal residues remain after harvest. Those that do are removed with the thick rind.

Mangoes. Mangoes are grown in Mexico, the Caribbean, and South America, where the dry climate discourages fungus and hand weeding is a common alternative to herbicides. In addition—repeat after us—mangoes are peeled before eating.

Sweet peas. They are protected by their pods.

Asparagus. The spears spring up so fast, there's little time for insects to attack.

Kiwifruit. Lacewings and parasitic wasps help control the pests that like to feed on kiwis.

Cabbage. The plant is sprayed, but the outer leaves that absorb pesticides are discarded before sale.

Eggplant. The eggplant has a slick surface that sheds chemicals easily.

Cantaloupe. Though the melons are sprayed with insecticides, we don't ingest them because the fruit is cut out of the thick rind before, well, you know.

Watermelon. The fruit has a thick protective rind that is not eaten.

Grapefruit. Although farmers often use fungicides to control green mold, most of the residues remain on the peel.

Sweet potato. The sweet potato has built-in defenses. If bitten, it oozes a milky-white sap that gums up insect mouthparts. Before they're sold, sweet potatoes are cured at warm temperatures and high humidity. This causes the skin to thicken, providing protection against damage and disease.

Honeydew melon. Honeydew may be washed in diluted chlorine during packing in order to ward off rot-inducing microbes. But—need we say it again?—you discard the rind before eating. See, you're an expert already.

Just remember that whether you opt for conventional or organic, you're better off eating more fruits and vegetables rather than less. And whatever produce you buy, wash or peel it before eating.

9

The Diabetes Promoter in
YOUR KITCHEN

Shake the salt habit now! Your life might depend on it. An easy way is with a 2-week salt cleanse. For 2 weeks, look at labels and recipes to monitor your salt intake. Aim to eat three 300-calorie meals per day, each with less than 300 milligrams of sodium. Avoid processed and packaged foods, as well as alcohol.

Which of the following is true of salt?

(a) It's addictive.

(b) It will make you fat.

(c) It will kill you.

(d) All of the above.

If you chose (d), you're right. Salt is one of the most dangerous ingredients in our food.

It's no secret that a high-sodium diet raises blood pressure, which in turn can cause heart attacks and strokes. But new studies show that salt is even more dangerous than we thought: Eating lots of salt might promote insulin resistance. Diabetes already puts you at greater risk of hypertension and heart disease—and a high salt intake only raises these risks. Plus, eating too much has been linked to osteoporosis, dementia, cancer, and other serious health problems. (See "The Silent Killer" on page 76.) Salt can also add inches to your waist.

Based on this research, the US government is revisiting its sodium guidelines. The new thinking: Adults should consume no more than 1,500 milligrams of sodium per day ($^2/_3$ teaspoon), down from the previous limit of less than 2,300 milligrams.

This adjustment means that Americans are seriously overdosing on salt, getting 3,436 milligrams a day—more than double the recommended amount.

Where's all that sodium coming from? The greatest concern isn't the flaky stuff you shake on at the table; it's the salt that's already in your food. The biggest culprits are processed and packaged foods, which load up on salt for flavor, color, and texture, and to prevent spoilage.

About 80 percent of the sodium in our diets is found in the premade crackers, cookies, cereals, soups, frozen dinners, and pasta sauces we eat at home. And that doesn't even cover fast-food and other restaurant meals.

Here's how a single ingredient with zero calories can be such a major cause of weight gain and killer health problems—and how you can sleuth out hidden sodium to protect your health.

Why Salt Is Addictive

Your body does need some sodium—to maintain the right balance of fluids, transmit nerve impulses, and contract and relax your muscles—but only about 500 milligrams per day. When you eat far more than that, your brain chemistry is altered.

Research shows that consuming salt triggers the release of dopamine, which is the neurotransmitter associated with the brain's pleasure center, making salty foods as addictive as nicotine and

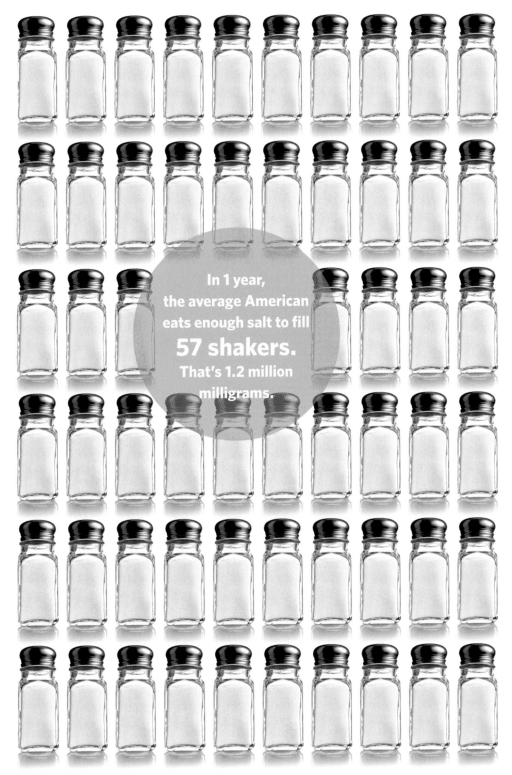

In 1 year,
the average American
eats enough salt to fill
57 shakers.
That's 1.2 million
milligrams.

THE SILENT KILLER

It's no longer just heart attacks and strokes you need to worry about if you eat too much salt. Evidence now connects sodium to other serious health problems, including the following.

Diabetes. Eating lots of salt might promote insulin resistance. Diabetes already puts you at greater risk of hypertension and heart disease, and a high salt intake raises these risks even more.

Cancer. Salted foods are linked to a 15 percent increase in cancer risk, according to a 2010 Japanese study. In other research, high salt intake has been associated with deaths from stomach cancer. Salty foods irritate the stomach lining, which can cause infection by *Helicobacter pylori,* bacteria that lead to stomach cancer.

Osteoporosis. High-salt diets have been shown to increase calcium loss, which weakens bone and leads, over time, to osteoporosis. A 2-year study of postmenopausal women connected a decrease in hip bone density to sodium intake.

Dementia. Hypertension might also affect your brain. Results of the 2010 Women's Health Initiative Memory Study, which took MRI scans of 1,400 women age 65 or older, revealed that those with high blood pressure had more abnormal brain lesions 8 years later. Other research shows that people with hypertension are up to 600 percent more likely to develop stroke-related dementia.

Sleep apnea. High blood pressure is a villain here, too. It is a vicious cycle: Sleep apnea causes sleep deprivation, which can increase blood pressure.

Kidney disease. Hypertension eventually damages blood vessels throughout your body, including the kidneys. The damage can be gradual: Symptoms might not occur until kidney function is less than 10 percent of normal.

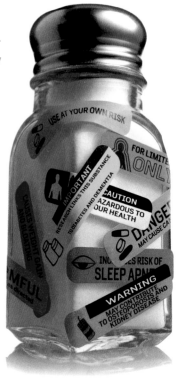

alcohol. Therefore, as with any addiction, eating salty foods makes you crave more. Because so many of them—such as french fries and fast-food sandwiches—are also high in fat and calories, OD'ing on salt packs on the pounds.

Loading up on salt also increases thirst. This wouldn't be an issue if we

There's Salt in That?

In a typical day, the sodium adds up fast—hidden in foods you probably didn't even know were salty.

Breakfast. 1 whole grain bagel *(490 milligrams)* with 2 tablespoons fat-free cream cheese *(211 milligrams)* and 6 ounces yogurt *(95 milligrams)* = 796 milligrams

Snack. 2 tablespoons peanut butter *(147 milligrams)* on 6 wheat crackers *(194 milligrams)* = 341 milligrams

Lunch. Sandwich with 2 slices low-salt turkey *(432 milligrams)*, 1 slice American cheese *(266 milligrams)*, and 2 teaspoons mustard *(114 milligrams)* in a flour tortilla *(490 milligrams)* with 1 dill pickle spear *(306 milligrams)* and 1 cup vegetable soup *(960 milligrams)* = 2,568 milligrams

Snack. 1 wheat pita *(340 milligrams)* with 2 tablespoons hummus *(114 milligrams)* = 454 milligrams

Dinner. $\frac{1}{2}$ cup pasta *(4 milligrams)* with $\frac{1}{2}$ cup jarred tomato sauce *(480 milligrams)* and 2 meatballs (232 milligrams), 1 slice garlic bread *(400 milligrams)*, and salad with reduced-fat ranch dressing *(336 milligrams)* = 1,452 milligrams

Dessert. Homemade apple crisp *(495 milligrams)* with $\frac{1}{2}$ cup vanilla ice cream *(53 milligrams)* and 2 tablespoons caramel sauce *(60 milligrams)* = 608 milligrams

Total: 6,219 milligrams, more than quadruple the daily recommended amount.

---

usually turned to water, but we don't. Research has found a close link between the consumption of salt and the intake of sugary beverages. (Diet sodas aren't the answer. They're full of sodium!)

Eating too much salt might cause weight gain in less noticeable ways, too—by changing how your body makes and metabolizes fat. Studies show that a high-salt diet boosts the production of insulin, the hormone that tells the body to store excess sugar as fat. Simply put, the more insulin you have, the more fat you store and the more weight you gain.

WANT SOME CHIPS WITH YOUR SALT?

Most regular chips have 160 to 180 milligrams of sodium per 1-ounce serving (about 15 chips). Watch out for flavored chips. The worst offenders of all: salt-and-vinegar chips.

The number of heart attacks that could be prevented each year if Americans consumed ½ teaspoon less of salt daily (1,163 milligrams of sodium), according to a report in the *New England Journal of Medicine.*

99,000

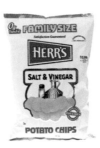

Herr's Salt & Vinegar:
340 milligrams

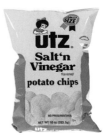

Utz Salt'n Vinegar:
270 milligrams

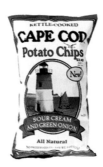

Cape Cod Sour Cream &
Green Onion: 220 milligrams

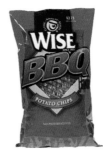

Wise BBQ:
210 milligrams

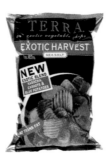

Terra Exotic Harvest Sea Salt:
160 milligrams

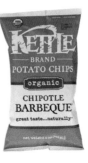

Kettle Brand Organic Chipotle Barbeque:
150 milligrams

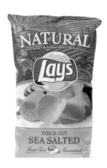

Lay's Natural Sea Salted:
150 milligrams

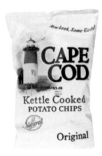

Cape Cod Original:
110 milligrams

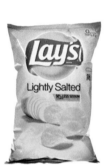

Lay's Lightly Salted:
90 milligrams

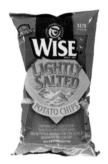

Wise Lightly Salted:
80 milligrams

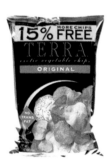

Terra Original:
50 milligrams

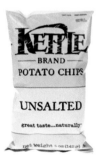

Kettle Brand Unsalted:
5 milligrams

3

LOSE

If you need to lose weight, consider that to be

WEIGHT

your best first step in managing your diabetes.

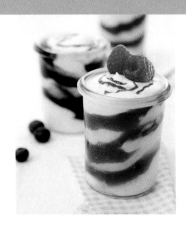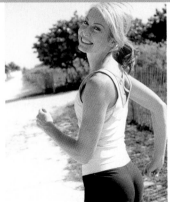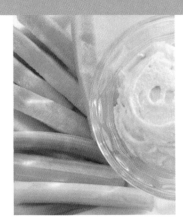

WEIGHT-LOSS
Breakthroughs

Weight and diabetes go together like chocolate and peanut butter. Experts say that if you have diabetes and you lose even just 5 to 10 percent of your weight, you'll significantly reduce your blood sugar. Here's the latest research into weight loss and its effect on diabetes.

CUT CALORIES AND WORK OUT

For optimal health, you must cut calories and work out—not one or the other. In a recent experiment, one group consumed 25 percent fewer calories; another cut calories by 12.5 percent and exercised off 12.5 percent (so the total calorie drop was equal). After 6 months, both groups lost weight, but only exercisers improved insulin sensitivity, blood pressure, and LDL cholesterol.

SHED FAT WITH SUNSHINE!

Treadmill burnout? Step outside for a bigger calorie burn. Research from Ohio State University found that walkers rated fresh-air exercise as more enjoyable and easier to maintain than treadmill routines. In another study, people got bigger boosts in physical and mental energy when they exercised outdoors compared with inside. And more daylight hours can naturally increase activity levels so you burn more calories. Research shows that 30 percent more women get active as the days get longer.

JUMP-START YOUR METABOLISM

Interval training is the speediest way to burn fat, and now new research shows that you don't have to push yourself until you're breathless to reap the benefits. According to Canadian scientists, exercisers who performed less intense intervals still increased key metabolism-revving enzymes by as much as 29 percent in just 6 workouts over 2 weeks. Best of all, it takes just 20 minutes a session, and you only have to push yourself to go hard for 8 minutes of it. Here's an easy way to do it.

20-MINUTE FAT-BURNING BLAST

It takes only 20 minutes of intervals to increase your natural calorie burn. Do the routine below every other day using your favorite cardiovascular activity, such as jogging or biking. For the "Push It" intervals, increase to a vigorous pace; you should be able to talk but need to take a breath after every few words. For the "Go Easy" portions, slow down to a comfortable pace.

The number of additional minutes spent exercising when outdoors versus inside.

24

Time	What to Do
0:00–2:59	Warm up at an easy pace.
3:00–3:59	Push It
4:00–4:59	Go Easy
5:00–18:59	Repeat minutes 3:00–4:59 seven more times.
19:00–20:00	Cool down at an easy pace.

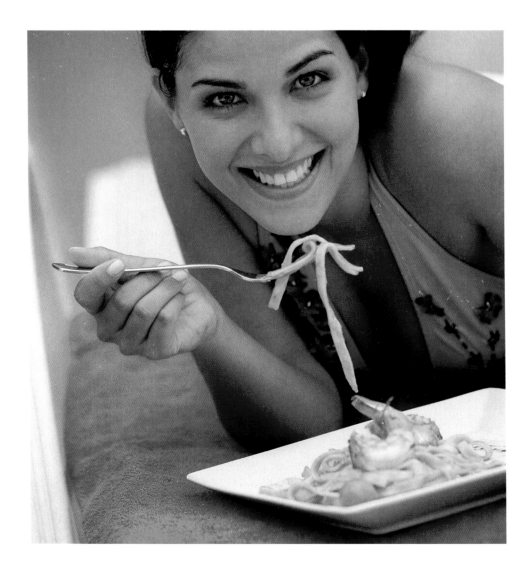

■ REEL IN HUNGER

Swedish researchers found that people who ate fish midday consumed 11 percent less at dinner—enough to lose 8 pounds in a year—compared with those who ate beef. Seafood's healthy fats may be the reason. "A meal high in omega-3 fatty acids can increase satiety for up to 2 hours," says Martha McKittrick, RD.

Here are three of our favorite hunger-busting lunch combos. Try one of these today!

Chunk light tuna + mixed greens + walnuts + balsamic vinaigrette

Salmon avocado roll + edamame + miso soup + green tea

Shrimp + soba noodles + broccoli + light soy sauce

SUPPLEMENT FOR SLIMNESS

New research shows the nutrients you need to stay healthy may also regulate hunger. Experts recommend getting them through food first, but because many women fall short, consider the supplements below for extra insurance.

CARB YOUR ENTHUSIASM!

When Australian researchers put people on reduced-calorie diets—one low-fat, the other low-carb—for 1 year, each group lost an average of 30 pounds. But the low-carb group (which cut out bread, pasta, and beans) felt more angry, depressed, and

Slimming Supplement	Research	Recommended Intake	Health Bonus
Vitamin D	People who have high vitamin D levels at the start of a diet lose more weight, suggests research presented at the Endocrine Society's annual meeting.	Get 1,000 IU through fatty fish and fortified cereal, juice, and dairy products or a vitamin D supplement daily.	Vitamin D fights cancer and helps your body absorb bone-building calcium.
Prebiotics	Overweight adults who took a prebiotic supplement lost an average of 2 pounds over 12 weeks compared with those on a placebo, found Canadian researchers.	Aim for 4 to 20 grams daily from foods such as garlic, onions, artichokes, and fortified yogurt, or supplements.	Prebiotics stimulate the growth of healthy bacteria (probiotics) in the gut to regulate digestion.
Calcium	When women deficient in calcium took 1,200 mg of calcium daily for 15 weeks, they lost four times as much weight as those who took a placebo.	Get 1,000–1,200 milligrams daily from low-fat dairy and leafy green vegetables or from a 500- or 600-milligram calcium carbonate or citrate supplement taken twice a day.	Calcium builds and maintains strong bones to prevent injury and osteoporosis.
Multivitamin	In a 15-week study, women who popped a daily multivitamin felt 45 percent less hungry than those who took a placebo.	Eat plenty of colorful fresh fruits and veggies, whole grains, and lean protein daily, and take a multivitamin that provides no more than 100 percent of your daily value for each nutrient.	The wide range of nutrients in multivitamins plays a critical part in immune function.

confused than the low-fat eaters. Carbohydrates help stimulate the production of mood-boosting serotonin. To lose weight and stay upbeat, eat a calorie-controlled diet with about 30 grams of healthy carbs, such as produce and whole grains, at every meal. (Talk with your diabetes doctor about the level of carbs that's best for you.)

■ TURN OFF THE TV

Here's a seriously easy way to cut calories: A recent *Journal of the American Medical Association* study found that when adults cut their viewing time in half, from $4^1/_2$ hours each day, they burned an extra 119 calories a day.

■ WATCH OUT FOR WEEKENDS

A sure way to derail a diet is to treat weekends like holidays, say researchers. They found that most people eat more on Saturdays and Sundays than on weekdays, with some taking in an average of 411 extra calories each day, which is enough to gain 12 pounds in a year. People consider the weekend a time to unwind and indulge, say researchers.

To avoid this weight trap, eat modest portions of your favorite foods, and up your activity by walking instead of driving to run errands, suggests cognitive therapist Judith S. Beck, PhD.

■ OUTSMART PMS CRAVINGS

Ever wonder why women are powerless before the charms of a brownie in the 2 weeks leading up to their periods? A new study reports that women eat 15 percent more calories during this phase of their cycle than they do during the rest. That's because their levels of appetite-suppressing estrogen decrease. Although their metabolism speeds up because of an increase in progesterone, this isn't enough to offset the extra calories most women consume.

Instead of bingeing on truffles and ice cream, head off cravings by pairing protein with good carbs at every meal, says Sari Greaves, RD, a spokesperson for the American Dietetic Association. For snacks, fat-free Greek yogurt sprinkled with berries, fruit with an ounce of cheese, or pretzels with hummus are healthy combos of protein and carbs, which reduce levels of hunger hormones so you don't have cravings. If nothing but chocolate will do, savor an ounce of quality dark.

10

Smart Food and Weight-Loss

STRATEGIES

Try these research-tested, expert-approved tips for people with diabetes.

O atmeal or toast and jelly? Pasta or broiled chicken and field greens? Fresh berries or a brownie sundae?

Ultimately, what you choose to eat—the little decisions you make in the kitchen, in the cafeteria line, or out to dinner—plays a major role in whether or not your blood sugar stays on an even keel, raising or lowering your risk for overweight, fatigue, and a host of major health problems.

Think of this chapter as a nutritional cheat sheet, with practical food wisdom that can help put you on the road to blood sugar control. Here, you'll find nutritional tips that reflect the current thinking on the relationship between diet and blood sugar, including high-protein diets, "good" and "bad" carbs, the glycemic index, fitting sweets into your diet, and much more. The more often you practice these recommendations, the more your blood sugar numbers stand to benefit.

Go on a Fiber Hunt

We'll skip the sermon about the health benefits of fruits and vegetables. And we've already talked a lot about fiber in Chapter 6. But we'd like to remind you that if you're trying to lose weight or control your blood sugar, fiber is your friend. A recent study showed that people with diabetes who ate 50 grams of fiber a day— particularly the soluble kind, found in foods like apples and oatmeal—were able to control their blood sugar better than those who ate far less.

Fiber is so important to health that the American Diabetes Association recently recommended that people who have diabetes or are at risk should strive for a whopping 50 grams a day. (Later in this chapter, we'll show you how to use a fiber supplement to help get there.) And the US Food and Nutrition Board recently set the first recommended daily intakes for healthy women and men. Consider these guidelines your minimum fiber requirement: Before age 50, men need 35 grams; women, 25 grams. After age 50, men need 30 grams; women, 31 grams.

Give Peas a Chance

And other beans, too. They're the highest-fiber foods you can find, with the exception of breakfast cereals made with wheat bran. High-fiber diets are linked to less diabetes and heart disease, and one study showed that as little as 3.4 ounces of beans a day helped people with diabetes manage their blood sugar levels. Beans are especially high in soluble fiber, which lowers cholesterol levels, and folate, which lowers homocysteine, another risk factor for heart disease.

Ideally, eat beans five or more times a week. They add protein and fiber to any dish and can be used in salads, stuffed baked potatoes, and veggie chili. Or puree

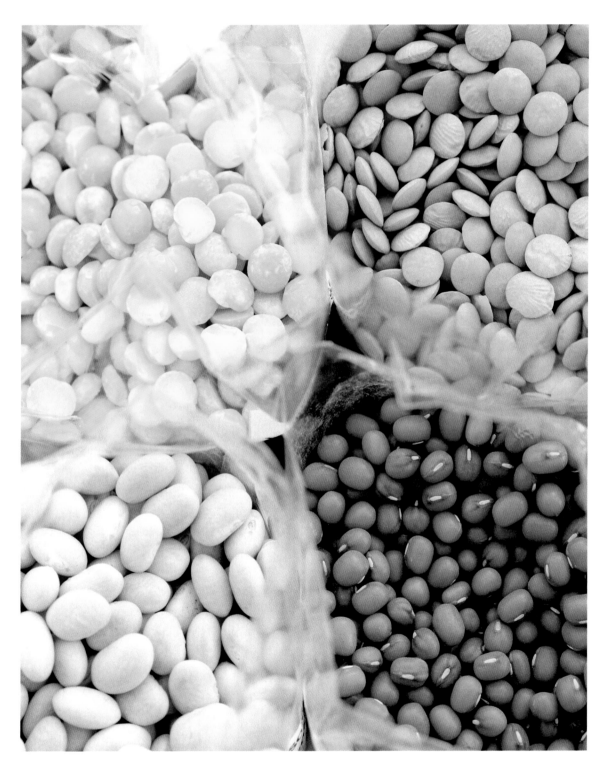

some to use as a sandwich spread. If you keep a variety of beans in your pantry, you'll always have the makings of a delicious, healthful dinner. If you use canned beans, remember to rinse them first because they're packed in a high-sodium liquid.

Instant bean soup is another great thing to have on hand. With instant bean soups, you have a heart-smart meal that's ready in about 6 minutes—and no dishes to wash. Good choices include Fantastic Foods Five Bean (240 calories, 1.5 grams fat, 12 grams fiber), Fantastic Foods Split Pea (220 calories, 1 gram fat, 9 grams fiber), and Knorr Hearty Lentil (220 calories, 2 grams fat, 8 grams fiber).

Go with the (Cereal) Grain

To your body, refined white flour is the same as sugar, making a diet high in white-flour foods the same as a high-sugar diet. Conversely, the evidence is accumulating that, besides cutting the risk of heart disease, stroke, and cancer, diets high in whole grains are linked to less diabetes.

In one of the most recent studies, Finnish researchers followed 2,286 men and 2,030 women ages 40 through 69 for 10 years. They found that those who ate the most fiber—not from fruits and vegetables but from cereal grains such as rolled oats, rye, barley, millet, and buckwheat—had a 61 percent lower risk of type 2 diabetes.

It's thought that cereal fiber may help fight type 2 diabetes in a couple of ways. Compared with simple carbohydrates such as white bread, fiber-rich carbs are digested and absorbed slowly, leading to less insulin demand. Also, insoluble fiber speeds through the intestines, leaving less time for carbohydrates to be absorbed. However, it's possible that other components in whole grains, such as lignans, tocotrienols, and phytic acids, could be responsible for the reduction in risk.

If you already eat whole wheat bread and need a change, try whole grain rye bread, which is what most of the cereal grain eaters in the Finnish study ate.

Select whole grain pastas—whole wheat, of course, but also those made with amaranth, quinoa, or buckwheat (including Japanese buckwheat noodles, known as soba noodles). You'll find them at upscale grocery stores or health food stores.

Keep to Your Fat Budget

Despite the long-running low-fat food craze in the United States, the amount of fat in our diets has actually been increasing.

On an 1,800-calorie diet with no more than 25 to 30 percent of calories coming from fat, we should get 50 to 60 grams of fat. And that should be 50 grams of good fat, like the types in olive and canola oils (monounsaturated fat) and fatty fish (omega-3 fatty acids).

You've probably already switched to

fat-free milk and low-fat dairy products. And you know you should trim visible fat from pork and beef and remove the skin from poultry.

It's a good idea to spread your fat throughout the day. A little fat helps you absorb fat-soluble nutrients from vegetables and fruit.

Use wine; lemon, orange, or tomato juice; herbs and spices; or broth instead of butter when cooking vegetables.

Switch from high-fat meats such as ribs and sausage (with 8 grams of fat per small serving) and higher-fat beef, pork, and lamb (with 5 grams per serving) to leaner cuts like skinless chicken or turkey breast, fish, lean pork, or USDA Choice or Select cuts of beef—all of which have about 3 grams of fat per serving or even less.

Flavor-test low-fat cheese. It doesn't taste like Styrofoam anymore, and ounce for ounce the low-fat stuff could save you 5 grams of fat per slice.

Get the Safest Fats from the Sea

For years, we've heard that fat causes heart attacks, high cholesterol, and weight gain. But we now know that certain types of fat actually protect us from high cholesterol, diabetes, and high blood pressure.

Omega-3 fatty acids, which we talked about in detail in Chapter 6, help lower bad LDL cholesterol, raise good HDL cholesterol, lower triglycerides (a type of blood fat), and may reduce the risk of blood clots. That's good news for everyone, but especially for folks with diabetes, who are more prone to heart disease.

Omega-3s aren't made by our bodies. We must get them from food, specifically fish and plants. Fish provides important omega-3 fats called EPA (eicosapentaenoic acid) and DHA (docosahexaenoic acid). Good sources include salmon, mackerel, sardines, herring, anchovies, rainbow trout, and bluefish.

Canned tuna is an easy, convenient source, but it's notorious for mercury contamination. Besides its well-known potential for damage to children's developing brains, accumulated mercury may impair adults' immune and reproductive systems and raise heart attack risk. Try canned salmon or mackerel instead, say Purdue University researchers who tested 272 cans of fish. They found that mercury levels averaged 45 ppb (parts per billion) in canned salmon and 55 ppb in mackerel, compared with as much as 340 ppb in tuna in oil.

If you love tuna, opt for cans labeled "chunk light tuna in water." Although they have less healthy omega-3 fats than salmon and mackerel, they averaged only 54 ppb of mercury.

According to the Environmental Working Group, which analyzed the mercury content of popular fish for its report, "Brain Food," the following fish are low enough in the toxic metal for even pregnant women to enjoy on a regular basis: croaker, farmed catfish, farmed trout, fish sticks, haddock, mid-Atlantic blue crab, shrimp, summer flounder, and wild Pacific salmon.

Ocean fish are less likely to contain high dioxin and PCB levels than freshwater fish, because ocean waters tend to be cleaner. Before cooking fish, remove the skin, fat, internal organs, tomalley from lobster, and mustard from crabs, all places where toxins are likely to accumulate. Avoid frying fish; it seals in chemical pollutants. Grilling and broiling allow toxins to drain away.

Say Nuts to Blood Sugar Problems

Whether you like to crunch on walnuts, pistachios, or almonds or spread nut butters on whole grain bread, you're in luck. Nuts are packed with protein, fiber, and good fats that keep you feeling full and satisfied for a long, long time. Nut eaters can cut their risk for diabetes by 20 to 30 percent, Harvard Medical School researchers have found. And this may be why: An amazing group of studies has found that people who eat nuts tend to eat less the rest of the day, automatically.

Still, nuts are packed with calories, so go easy. Avoid tagalong bad fats. Pass up snack bags of flavored nuts if the list of ingredients includes "partially hydrogenated oils"—shorthand for trans fats.

Cup a snack in your palm. A palmful of nuts is, in general, 1 ounce—the perfect snack size. Prefer to count 'em out? An ounce equals 14 walnut halves, 18 cashews, 20 pecan halves, 50 dry-roasted pistachios, 10 to 20 macadamia nuts (depending on size), or 24 filberts.

Discover Plate Power

Unless you've been living underground the past few years, you know that protein has made a comeback and carbohydrates have lost favor. It's understandable that you might be tempted to jump on the pro-protein bandwagon—if you haven't already.

Don't do it. There's nothing wrong with carbohydrates such as beans, whole grain cereal, or apples. It's highly processed carbs like cookies and cake that pack on the pounds.

To calculate your protein and carbohydrate needs, simply follow the "plate rule."

- Fill half your plate with vegetables and/or fruits.
- Fill the remainder with roughly equal amounts of starch and a high-protein food.

Eat this way, and you can watch the weight come off—while you lower your risk of diabetes, cancer, and other diseases.

Go on Portion Patrol

Most restaurants serve bowls of pasta as deep as mixing bowls or sandwiches thicker than a paperback. We pile our plates high at home, too. That's why many of us find it difficult to trim our waistlines. Mammoth portions aren't just adding extra calories to our diets. Chances are, they're also adding more fat, sugar, and salt.

One solution: Start reading the serving sizes on food labels. More often than not, the package of chips you have with lunch contains 2 or $2^1/_2$ servings, not 1.

Also, learn what one serving of a particular food really looks like. For example, one serving of meat is $3^1/_2$ ounces and fits in the palm of your hand; one serving of whole grain pasta is $1/_2$ cup and the size of a tennis ball.

Give Trans Fats the Boot

At last! Starting in 2006, food labels list levels of unhealthy trans fats, the "Frankenfat" that gunks up arteries and raises heart disease risk. But zero plus zero doesn't always equal zero. New FDA labeling rules allow foods with less than 0.5 gram of trans fats per serving to claim "zero" grams of trans fats on their labels.

Under these guidelines, a food with 0.4 gram of trans fats can be listed as having zero trans fats. That means that Americans who consume three or four servings of these foods a day will unwittingly have eaten an extra gram or two of trans fats. That's important, because trans fats, like saturated fats, can raise the risk of heart disease as they increase levels of bad LDL cholesterol.

Currently, the FDA estimates that Americans consume an average 5.8 grams of trans fats per day. Barbara Schneeman, director of the Office of Nutritional Products, Labeling, and Dietary Supplements for the FDA, says the reason the FDA is allowing foods under 0.5 gram of trans fats to be rounded down to zero is that current detection methods for trans fats aren't very reliable below 0.5 gram.

So, what's a concerned consumer to do? "If you see a food with zero trans fat, check the ingredient list for the words 'partially hydrogenated.' If you see 'partially hydrogenated,' that means the product contains some trans fats," advises nutritionist Samantha Heller from New York University Langone Medical Center.

The FDA adds that products with shortening or hydrogenated oils in their ingredient lists also contain some trans fats, and the higher up the list you find those items, the greater the amount of trans fats the product contains.

Trans fats are created when liquid oils are transformed into solids, a process called hydrogenation. They're prevalent in many processed foods because they add to a product's shelf life and increase flavor stability. Heller says that most foods containing trans fats are foods you should eat in moderation, including deep-fried restaurant foods, doughnuts, cookies, cakes, and muffins.

Get the Salt Out

We believe in moderation when it comes to salt. So does Myron Weinberger, MD, director of the Hypertension Research Center at Indiana University School of Medicine in Indianapolis. "You don't need to drastically cut back on salt," he explains. Adults should consume no more than 1,500 milligrams a day—$^2/_3$ teaspoon total from all sources. The average American gets about 3,400 milligrams of sodium a day, so that means cutting our usual intake by about half.

Cutting back can help lower high blood pressure and, if your blood pressure is normal now, cut your risk for developing it later in life. (High blood pressure often accompanies metabolic syndrome, prediabetes, and diabetes.) An easy way to dial down the sodium by 25 percent is by using kosher or coarse salt instead—the coarse granules don't pack as tightly into a measuring spoon.

Think Before You Drink

If you have type 2 diabetes, it's okay to drink alcoholic beverages in moderation as long as your blood sugar is under control. The key is moderation: one drink a day for women, two for men. A drink is defined as one 4-ounce glass of wine, one 12-ounce bottle of beer, or a drink made with $1^1/_2$ ounces of distilled liquor. Heavier drinking can worsen the complications of diabetes.

Be Picky about Sugar-Free Foods

Some foods labeled "sugar-free" or "no sugar added" may actually raise your blood sugar nearly as much as the regular version. That's because some sugar-free cookies, cakes, or other sweet treats may contain nearly as many carbohydrates as the real sugar-laden thing. Adding insult to injury, they might also pack nearly as many calories.

The fact is, not all sugar substitutes are the same—yet another reason to scrutinize a food's Nutrition Facts label. Here's what you should know about them.

Sugar alcohols. Many sugar-free foods contain sugar alcohols such as sorbitol or mannitol. These carbohydrate-based ingredients contain about half the calories of regular carbs, about 2 per gram. By law, they don't have to be counted as sugars on the Nutrition Facts labels, but they still add to the bottom-line carb count. Verdict: Many diabetes experts say these foods aren't of much benefit for diabetes control. You're better off with a small portion of the real thing.

Sugar substitutes. FDA-approved sugar substitutes such as acesulfame-K (Sweet One), aspartame (NutraSweet), and sucralose (Splenda) contain no calories or carbohydrates. Foods sweetened with them may contain no calories (like diet soda), or they might contain some calories and carbohydrates from other ingredients (like hot cocoa mix).

Of all the artificial sweeteners, Splenda has drawn the least amount of controversy over its safety. It's one of the most tested sugar substitutes, showing no harmful effects in more than 100 studies on humans and animals. Unlike some sugar substitutes, you can bake with Splenda, which is made from sugar but has no calories. For tips on how to bake with Splenda, as well as some delicious recipes, go to www.splenda.com.

Verdict: Check the carb content of any food sweetened with sugar substitutes. They might be a lower-carb way to enjoy a little treat.

Choose Chocolate That Loves Your Heart

Adore chocolate? Fear heart disease? Start celebrating. Just 1 ounce of one brand of chocolate has more than twice the heart-healthy antioxidant punch of red wine or other dark chocolate.

Dove Dark, made by Mars, contains Cocoapro cocoa, a proprietary, specially processed cocoa that contains superhigh levels of antioxidant flavonoids called flavanols—so high that Dove Dark is used in medical research. Studies have shown that people with high blood levels of flavonoids have lower risk of type 2 diabetes and heart disease.

Researchers at the University of California, Davis, compared the effects of $1\frac{1}{3}$ ounces of high-flavanol Dove Dark chocolate with the same amount of low-flavanol dark chocolate on 10 healthy people. Only the Dove Dark reduced LDL oxidation and boosted antioxidant levels and HDL concentrations in the blood.

In the test tube, Cocoapro cocoa reduces blood clotting. It may also stabilize arterial plaque, making it less likely to travel and cause a stroke or heart attack. This effect is similar to that of aspirin. Some of the procyanidins in Cocoapro trigger the production of nitric oxide, which helps keep arteries flexible and increases blood flow.

The chocolates with the highest cocoa content have the highest flavanol content. Two with superior levels of flavanol:

- El Rey Gran Saman Dark Chocolate, 1.4 ounces, 70 percent cocoa, 190 calories, 15 grams fat

- Scharffen Berger Bittersweet, 1-ounce bar, 70 percent cocoa, 170 calories, 11 grams fat

Several studies in animals and humans have shown the heart-healthy effects of chocolate's antioxidants, which is a boon for people with type 2 diabetes, who are at higher risk for heart disease. One of these studies, led by Penny Kris-Etherton, PhD, RD, distinguished professor of nutrition at Pennsylvania State University in

University Park, found that people who ate a diet rich in cocoa powder and dark chocolate had lower oxidation levels of bad LDL cholesterol, higher blood antioxidant levels, and 4 percent higher levels of good HDL cholesterol.

Eat Early and Often

If you commonly skip breakfast, skimp on lunch, gorge on a lumberjack-size dinner, and engage in lots of noshing in the hours before bed, it's likely that you're sending your blood sugar on a wild roller-coaster ride. Blood sugar plummets in response to the lack of food during the day and surges in response to that huge evening meal. Because the skip-and-gorge way of eating encourages overeating, it's not so good for your waistline, either.

There's a better way to control your blood sugar while you watch your calories and portion sizes: Consider having four to six minimeals of about 250 calories throughout your day rather than eating three big meals a day.

"By eating smaller, more frequent meals, with the correct proportions of proteins, fats, and carbohydrates, you may be manipulating your hormones in favor of reaching the weight you want," says Geoffrey Redmond, MD, director of the Hormone Center of New York in New York City and author of *The Good News about Women's Hormones.*

The minimeal strategy helps keep your blood sugar levels in check through what's known as the second-meal effect: The closer one small meal is to the next, the less your glucose levels will soar, which means lower insulin on a regular basis.

Minimeals might also help keep your weight in check, especially if you're a woman in midlife. In a study conducted at Tufts University in Boston, when healthy older women (average age 72) ate 500- and 1,000-calorie meals, their blood sugar and insulin levels remained high for up to 5 hours. (In young women, those levels quickly returned to normal.) But after 250-calorie meals, the older women's blood sugar and insulin did what they're supposed to do—rise, and then return rapidly to normal.

Just make sure your meals are truly mini, however. Calories from small, frequent snacks and meals can add up fast, even if you're skipping fat- and sugar-laden snacks and opting for healthier fare.

Beef Up Your Diet—Sensibly

Too much fat. Too many calories. A shortcut to heart disease. Many health-conscious people have drastically curtailed their intake of red meat, but there's no reason to forgo meat if you go lean. In addition to being a very good source of protein, lean beef is an excellent source of vitamin B_{12} and a good source of vitamin B_6, which the body needs to convert the potentially heart-threatening chemical homocysteine into more benign molecules. Lean red meat is also packed with zinc, a mineral women often lack. One 3-ounce serving of beef has as much zinc as $5^1/_2$ chicken breasts. And one-third of the saturated fat in beef is stearic acid, a fatty acid that has a neutral effect on blood cholesterol levels.

The steaks, burgers, and roasts in today's supermarkets are leaner than ever. To eat beef sensibly, look for the words "lean" or "extra lean" on the label; these cuts have 4.5 grams or less of saturated fat and 5 to 10 grams of total fat per serving. Or look for these lean cuts: bottom, eye, or top round; round tip; top sirloin; top loin; or tenderloin.

Just Say Moo

Extra body fat and too little exercise lull your body into resisting the efforts of insulin, the hormone that sends blood sugar into your cells.

Now researchers say that even if you're overweight, choosing more low-fat dairy products—such as a glass of 1% milk or a smoothie made with low-fat yogurt instead of a soda—could help preserve your cells' insulin sensitivity and cut short the first steps on the road to diabetes.

In a 10-year study of 3,000 people, those who were overweight but consumed lots of dairy were 70 percent less likely than dairy avoiders to develop insulin resistance. "The lactose, protein, and fat in milk all have the potential to improve blood sugar," says researcher

Mark A. Pereira, PhD, of the University of Minnesota. "Milk sugar [lactose] is converted to blood sugar at a relatively slow rate, which is good for blood sugar control and reducing insulin levels. Protein helps fill you up. And fat may keep you feeling satisfied, too." Nutrients in dairy products, including calcium, magnesium, and potassium, also help.

To fight diabetes with dairy, aim for at least two servings of low-fat dairy foods daily. Each serving cuts the odds of insulin resistance by 20 percent. Make smart switches. Have dairy products instead of high-carbohydrate, low-fiber snacks such as soda, sweets, or fast food.

Add a Little Spice to Your Day

Cinnamon does more than give a spicy lift to food: It also helps regulate blood sugar.

Cinnamon stimulates the production of glucose-burning enzymes and increases the effectiveness of insulin, says Richard A. Anderson, PhD, a chemist at the USDA Beltsville Human Nutrition Research Center in Maryland. Taking between $1/_4$ and 1 teaspoon of cinnamon—the same kind you buy at the supermarket—every day helps control blood sugar levels.

Dr. Anderson's search for a natural way to keep blood sugar levels normal began more than a decade ago, when he and his co-workers tested plants and spices used in folk medicine. They found that a few spices, especially cinnamon, made fat cells much more responsive to insulin, the hormone that regulates sugar metabolism and thus controls the level of glucose in the blood.

Dr. Anderson and his colleagues found that the most active compound in cinnamon is methylhydroxy chalcone polymer (MHCP), which increased glucose metabolism by about 20 times in test-tube studies.

MHCP also prevented the formation of damaging free radicals. "That could be an important side benefit," notes Dr. Anderson. "Other studies have shown that antioxidant supplements can reduce or slow the progression of various complications of diabetes."

Experiment with adding cinnamon to foods such as meat loaf or oatmeal, suggests Dr. Anderson. His favorite way is to boil a cinnamon stick in water for tea. "Just one stick gives you the same benefit as 1 teaspoon of ground cinnamon."

Enjoy a Spot of Tea

Love your cup of morning or afternoon Earl Grey or green tea? Now you can love it even more: Common teas boost insulin activity more than fifteenfold, according to studies conducted by the USDA.

Researchers at the USDA Beltsville Human Nutrition Research Center analyzed a variety of herbs, spices, and plants to see if they had any beneficial effect on insulin. They tested fat cells taken from rats—which they grew in test tubes—and "fed" the cells mildly radioactive sugar,

insulin, and various tea extracts. (Radioactive sugar was easy to track.)

The result: Black, green, and oolong teas—both caffeinated and noncaffeinated—enhanced insulin activity the most. Herbal teas did not. Further, adding whole, fat-free, or soy milk or nondairy creamer seemed to dampen the tea's beneficial effect on insulin.

The chemical in tea that appears to enhance insulin the most is called epigallocatechin gallate (EGCG). When green tea is oxidized into oolong and black tea, EGCG forms other compounds, called polyphenols, which are also strong antioxidants.

This insulin-boosting activity also might explain why tea seems to help prevent heart disease and high blood pressure. Medical investigators think that high blood sugar damages blood vessels and that increasing insulin activity lowers blood sugar levels.

You can drink from one to five cups of green, black, or oolong tea daily. If caffeine makes you jittery or you have a medical condition that prevents you from taking caffeine, feel free to drink the decaffeinated variety.

By the way, if you use tea bags and dunk the bag up and down while the tea brews, you get a huge bonus: The movement causes the tea to release vastly more of its polyphenols. In studies, tea bags dunked continuously for 3 minutes released five times more. If you use loose leaf tea, you don't need to dunk; tea leaves release more of their polyphenols whether or not they get a workout.

Unwrap the Right Bar

What's not to love about snack bars? They're convenient. They travel well. They don't spoil or go stale. They taste great. And now, several companies are manufacturing bars formulated just for people with high blood sugar.

Among these specialty bars are ChoiceDM Nutrition Bar, ExtendBar, and Glucerna. In one study, people with diabetes ate a ChoiceDM Nutrition Bar with slow-digesting carbohydrates and an energy bar with standard carbs. One hour after they ate the ChoiceDM bar, their insulin levels were 28 percent lower and their blood glucose was 16 percent lower than after the energy bar. (Elevated insulin and blood glucose levels are responsible for the damage diabetes can do.)

Many of these bars contain resistant starch, which is a type of carbohydrate that is digested and absorbed by the body at a slower rate. That means they don't raise blood glucose levels as quickly as other carbohydrate sources. The slow absorption also allows glucose to continue entering the bloodstream for a long time. This can help prevent hypoglycemia, especially in the middle of the night, when most of the carbohydrates consumed in a bedtime snack would normally be used up. As a bonus, these bars also contain vitamins, minerals, and fiber.

The bars are ideal almost anytime, including before, during, or after exercise; as a snack; or as part of a quick meal when your schedule hits a snag and you can't eat a meal at the usual time.

If you want to try these bars, talk to your doctor first about fitting them into your meal plan. Once you have her okay, test your blood sugar levels frequently—before and after eating bars and in the morning—to see how you're responding to a particular bar.

One more thing: Don't use these bars to treat hypoglycemia. They might not raise blood glucose levels as quickly as the glucose in a glass of juice or a piece of hard candy.

Brighten Up Breakfast

Researchers at the National Weight Control Registry have been studying 3,000 people who've lost at least 30 pounds and kept it off for a year or more, looking for patterns to explain their success. One common trait is that 80 percent eat breakfast every day.

But there's even better news. You can eat virtually anything you want for your morning meal as long as it's healthy, from a bowl of soup to a healthy sandwich on whole grain bread.

Log On, Lose Weight

The research is clear: People who track their daily intake of calories and nutrients find it easier to manage their weight and prevent weight gain. That's a good reason to take advantage of the many free diet analysis tools on the Internet.

Below, you'll find some of the most reliable sites that can help you analyze and track your dietary intake and, in many cases, your physical activity. Most were cited in a report published in the *Journal of the American Dietetic Association*.

www. cnpp.usda.gov. Includes the popular Interactive Healthy Eating Index, developed by the USDA Center for Nutrition Policy and Promotion. Along with the ability to analyze food composition, this site will help you see how your daily diet stacks up against national standards.

www.fitday.com. One of the most popular sites, Fitday allows you to track your food intake as well as your physical activity. You can also monitor your personal diet and exercise goals. This site offers as many as or more features than some pay sites.

www.nutritiondataself.com. This freebie site will give you a complete nutritional analysis of a single food or let you compare the attributes of several foods. In addition, it can help you track your calorie consumption and even analyze and suggest improvements to your favorite recipes.

www.dietsite.com. This program includes a database of 5,600 foods to help in analyzing diets and recipes. Users can log on to track their food intake over several days and compare it to recommended daily intakes. This site also features nutrition news, message boards, and nutrition advice provided by a registered dietitian.

Snack on Stomach-Satisfying Protein

Healthy, planned snacking can prevent you from piling too much food on your plate for lunch and dinner. While many dieters turn to low-fat popcorn, pretzels, crackers, or sweets at snack time, research suggests that this carbohydrate load may be sabotaging weight loss. French researchers found that high-protein snacks keep you full longer and might reduce the amount you eat at your next meal.

"High-carbohydrate snackers got hungry as quickly as subjects who had no snack at all," says study author Jeanine Louis-Sylvestre, PhD. "But protein eaters, who snacked on chicken, stayed full nearly 40 minutes longer." Since it takes longer for protein to break down, you stay satisfied longer. (Note: Snackers ate 200-calorie snacks.)

Most of us don't think of chicken as a snack, but 2 ounces pack a powerful protein punch. Try prebaked chicken strips, (38 grams protein, 180 calories); a 3-ounce can of white chicken (14 grams protein, 70 calories); or a fast-food grilled chicken sandwich, minus the bun, mayo, and toppings (28 grams protein, 160 calories). Other options: 1 cup of low-fat cottage cheese (28 grams protein, 164 calories) or two string cheese sticks (14 grams protein, 160 calories).

Don't Believe Your Eyes

In a surprising Swedish study, volunteers ate 22 percent less food when they were blindfolded yet reported that they felt just as full as usual. To harness this in-the-dark eating experience, you could travel to a trendy Parisian restaurant, *Dans Le Noir* (In the Dark), where patrons eat in total darkness. Or simply pay more attention to your other senses when you sit down to a good bowl of homemade chicken noodle soup at your kitchen table.

Here are some practical ways to tune in to your body's hunger and satisfaction cues—and eat less.

- Clear the table. Place the mail and other clutter elsewhere. Set out just the dinnerware and a candle or simple flower centerpiece.

- Avoid distractions. Don't watch TV or read while you dine. When you do other things while you eat, you're less likely to notice when you're comfortably full.

- Go solo. Eating alone allows you to focus. If that's not practical, limit your number of dinner companions.

- Serve individual courses. Eat your salad first, then have your entrée. Leave the extras on the stove, and put only the food you're eating on the table. This will stretch out your meal so you'll recognize sooner when you've had enough.

- Close your eyes (for the first few bites). Taste what you're eating.

- Use the "Five Ds." When you catch yourself eating more than you'd like, follow these steps.

1. Determine what's going on.

2. Delay your response by figuring out what's driving your urge to eat: Anger? Boredom? Loneliness?

3. Distract yourself for at least 10 minutes.

4. Distance yourself from temptation. Throw away the chips. Heck, bury them in the garbage if you have to.

5. Decide how you'll handle the situation: Will you stop eating or continue? It's okay to keep going, as long as you make a conscious choice to continue rather than remain helplessly out of control.

De-Fang Your Diet Saboteurs

Want to bring out the worst in people? Lose weight. The problem usually starts because you're in change mode (and darned happy to be there), but your friends and family aren't. In fact, in one survey, 24,000 overweight women reported that losing weight created problems in their relationships that regaining the weight would have resolved.

"Rarely would a real friend malevolently undermine your diet," says nutrition professor Audrey Cross, PhD, of Rutgers University in New Brunswick, New Jersey. "They just do unconscious things to keep the relationship the way it was."

There are lots of reasons why. Perhaps they feel guilty, or maybe they miss sharing food with you. Whatever the reason, you need to protect yourself from these often well-meaning saboteurs. Below are some healthier, lower-calorie options when friends or family are enticing you.

Don't Let "Fattitudes" Weigh You Down

It's true that diabetes and other conditions that affect your blood sugar, like polycystic ovary syndrome (PCOS) for women, can make it more difficult to lose those stubborn pounds. But don't give up and let your good intentions be undermined by bad attitudes. To stay the course, adjust these common mental monkey wrenches.

The "fattitude": "I was born to be fat."

The reality: A USDA study found that women who think their gene pools preordain their jean sizes were more likely to be heavy. "Genes do have an impact on weight," says Thomas Wadden, PhD, director of the Weight and Eating Disorders Program at the University of Pennsylvania in Philadelphia. "But it's your environment that ultimately determines how fat you become."

The attitude adjustment: "The food and lifestyle choices I make shape my shape."

The "fattitude": "I won't be a happy or

Instead of...	Try...
Scarfing down wings and blue cheese with friends	Going to a restaurant where they can still get wings and you can get healthier food
Ordering dessert	Agreeing to share, then having only a forkful or two and spending lots of time raving about how wonderful it is
A 2-hour lunch	Eating a quick lunch, then shopping or taking a walk
Girls' night out at a restaurant or bar	Going to a spa for a manicure and pedicure; you can talk your heads off and have a great time
Guys' night out	Playing a pickup basketball game at the gym
Sharing a candy bar with your partner	Dipping strawberries in chocolate, giving his-and-her foot rubs, bringing home jewelry or playoff tickets

even a healthy person until I lose lots of weight."

The reality: "I see patients who set out wanting to lose 35 percent of their initial weight," says Dr. Wadden. "Then they're surprised at how good a 10 percent loss feels." They're probably basking in the glow of better health. One study proved that just a 7 percent weight loss and increased physical activity can delay or even prevent type 2 diabetes in high-risk people—and it did it so dramatically that the study ended a year early.

The attitude adjustment: "I'll be happier and healthier if I lose just 10 to 15 pounds."

The "fattitude": "I don't eat out much."

The reality: Maybe not in the special occasion sense, but every cafeteria lunch, take-out dinner, and vending machine snack still counts as food you don't cook at home. And that's dangerous because, for too many of us, dining out is tantamount to pigging out.

The attitude adjustment: "How many calories are hiding in this meal I didn't make?"

Use Your Cooking Style to Eat Healthier

When 440 great home cooks took a personality test devised by food science researchers, most fell into one of five "kitchen types." Some dished out comfort food. Others were trendsetters. Still others followed recipes to the letter.

Which of the gourmets listed below do you resemble?

Your kitchen type—innovative. You try new ingredients, new combinations, and new ways of cooking. Follow every step of a recipe? Never!

Cooking style: Like Jamie Oliver, the Naked Chef, you're a trendsetter who serves custard as part of the main meal and decorates the salad with edible flowers. You can cook healthy, but it's never a goal.

Healthy makeover: Add exotic, sophisticated ingredients packed with flavor and nutrition. Don't forget about farm-stand treasures such as heirloom veggies and those featured in ethnic cuisines such as collard greens.

Your kitchen type—giving. Your meals are welcoming and nurturing. Think Betty Crocker or TV's *Two Fat Ladies.*

Cooking style: Cozy, creamy delights such as yummy mac and cheese.

Healthy makeover: Go for small changes. Try roasted chicken instead of fried or baked potatoes with low-fat sour cream.

Your kitchen type—competitive. Ever flamboyant, you cook to impress.

Cooking style: Like Emeril Lagasse, you savor challenging recipes, leaping on trends and mastering them—whether the dishes are healthy or not.

Healthy makeover: Up your "oh, wow" factor by adding unique healthy ingredients such as gooseberries or Asian winter melon to perk up a boring meal.

Your kitchen type—methodical. You're a weekend Julia Child, following recipes to a T—with great results.

Cooking style: You use family recipes and those from gourmet magazines.

Healthy makeover: Prowl the cookbook section of your local bookstore and select a healthy cookbook you'd normally never buy but that intrigues you. Then let yourself go!

Supplement Your Fiber Intake

If you just can't manage to eat the recommended nine servings of fruits and vegetables a day, or if you're trying to eat the American Diabetes Association's recently recommended 50 grams of fiber per day, consider taking a fiber supplement. In particular, people with diabetes or high cholesterol can benefit from extra fiber, says James W. Anderson, MD, professor of medicine and clinical nutrition at the University of Kentucky and chief of the endocrine-metabolic section at the Veterans Affairs Medical Center, both in Lexington.

Selecting a fiber supplement from the dozens on the shelves seems like a daunting task, but Dr. Anderson cuts down your choices. To improve cholesterol and blood sugar levels, reach for a soluble-fiber supplement like psyllium husk, such as that found in Metamucil products.

Another choice is to opt for guar gum, a natural fiber ingredient in Benefiber. It dissolves into drinks and soft foods with no gritty feel or strange flavor. Dr. Anderson, however, favors psyllium husk because it is the most extensively studied fiber on the market.

Many dietitians recommend powdered supplements, such as the types made from psyllium or beta-glucan, which you mix into a glass of water. That way, you're sure to have the water your body needs to feel comfortable with so much extra fiber on board.

When you first boost your intake, intestinal bacteria will interact with the fiber to cause excess gas and bloating. To minimize discomfort, start with a low dose and slowly work your way up. Or try Citrucel, which contains methylcellulose, a soluble fiber that doesn't interact with the bacteria. No interaction means no unwanted side effects.

When you take fiber supplements, it's crucial to drink plenty of water throughout the day. Take the majority of fiber products with an 8-ounce glass of water. Start with a single dose, and work up to twice daily if needed. Fiber supplements won't block absorption of most drugs, but to be safe take them 2 hours before or after your medication, especially any for the heart or blood pressure, says Dr. Anderson.

11

Your Friend, the Scale

(REALLY!)

If you're trying to drop pounds, the scale is one of your most powerful allies. Here's how to use it, and keep your self-esteem intact.

For years, many experts recommended tossing your scale. That was good advice when you consider the emotional whiplash that weighing yourself can cause. As the number goes down, your confidence goes up, but a gain of even a pound can easily ruin your day.

It's time to end the love-hate relationship with your scale. A review of a dozen studies tracking more than 16,000 dieters provides indisputable evidence that the bathroom scale is one of the most effective tools for losing weight and preventing pounds from creeping on. A whopping 75 percent of members of the National Weight Control Registry—men and women who have lost at least 30 pounds and kept it off—weigh themselves at least once a week.

Here are five surprising facts that will help you make peace with your scale, and use it to your weight-loss advantage.

The More You Weigh Yourself, the More You Lose

Out of sight, out of mind simply doesn't work. In one study, daily weighers dropped twice as many pounds as weekly weighers—12 pounds versus 6, possibly because it was a regular reminder to stay on track. Meanwhile, dieters who avoided the scale altogether gained 4 pounds. And despite the common belief that focusing on weight makes women feel bad about themselves, scientists have found that tracking your weight can actually improve your mood by giving you a sense of control.

Tip. Weigh yourself daily. (More than

that isn't really meaningful, as you'll see in "The Scale Diary" on page 108.)

A Cheaper Model Is Better

You can spend hundreds on a high-tech scale that also estimates your body fat percentage and more through a series of mathematical algorithms, but you're just getting another number to worry about that's possibly less accurate than your weight.

"I avoid scales that measure body fat, because there are so many inaccuracies based on fluctuations in how much water you drink," says exercise physiologist Kara Mohr, PhD, who's done extensive scientific research on weight loss.

Tip. Buy a basic digital scale that displays weight to the nearest $1/2$ or $2/10$ pound to minimize fluctuations.

Weight Can Fluctuate 5 Pounds in 24 Hours

The biggest culprit is water (and water in the food you eat). The calories in a liter of soda would add about $1/10$ pound if you didn't burn them off, but step on the scale immediately after drinking it and you'll be up more than 2 pounds. Go to the bathroom and you'll likely drop 1 to $1 1/2$ pounds.

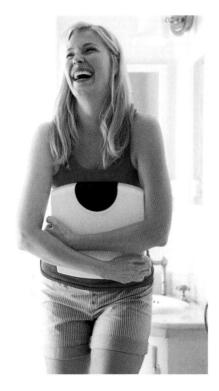

and focus on the pattern over time. The number may go up and down from one day to the next, but the overall direction month to month should be down if you're trying to lose weight. If you see an upward trend, it's time to take action.

You Can Lose Inches without Weighing Less

In a recent study from the University of California, Berkeley, women in their mid-fifties followed a 12-week cycling routine while eating a diet designed to maintain their weight. The result: One 56-year-old lost just 1 pound but dropped two sizes, thanks to a 7 percent decrease in body fat. She replaced about 4 pounds of fat with 4 pounds of muscle. Pound for pound, muscle is firmer and denser, and it takes up about one-third the space of fat. But don't assume your scale is stuck because of your new muscle. It takes about a

You even lose water weight—about 2 pounds a day—just by breathing and sweating. Day-to-day fluctuations can be the result of a high-sodium meal or your level of hydration, while your menstrual cycle can cause changes all month long. "It's important to keep the bigger picture in mind," says Dr. Mohr. No one meal or single splurge will move the scale's needle in a lasting way unless it becomes a habit. However, a difference of 100 calories at every meal could add up to more than 30 pounds in a year—in either direction.

Tip. Weigh yourself at the same time each day, first thing in the morning after using the bathroom and getting undressed, to avoid factors like water weight and clothing. Track your results,

WE TRIED IT! THE NUMBERLESS SCALE

Mary Lou's Weigh Platform (notice it's not even called a scale) secretly records your starting point, then simply tells you how much you're up or down each day. And Olympic gymnast Mary Lou Retton, who created the device, cheers you on with music, applause, and healthy tips. "You can't help but smile or even do a little dance," our tester said. "Not the usual reaction to weighing yourself!" ($49.95; marylousweigh.com)

month of strength training to add a single pound of muscle, on average, according to Wayne Westcott, PhD, author of *Get Stronger, Feel Younger*.

Tip. Track other markers such as the size of your waist and thighs (using a tape measure), how your clothes fit, or how much energy you have—and celebrate those successes.

Where You Put Your Scale Matters

In most cases, your bathroom floor will work just fine, but if the floor is textured or the grout creates an uneven surface, the readout might be off. Bath mats or carpet can absorb some of your weight, throwing off the scale's sensors and decreasing your weight by 20 pounds or more, said Keith Erickson, spokesperson for Tanita scales. Some higher-end scales come with carpet feet to accommodate the inconsistencies, but our tester still found a several-pound discrepancy.

Tip. Weigh yourself in the same spot every day.

Even if it's off by a few pounds, you'll still be able to see changes over time. For the most accurate reading, place your scale on a bare floor that's hard, flat, and level. You can test the scale's accuracy by weighing an object whose weight you know, like a dumbbell.

The Scale Diary

Don't let the number determine your self-worth! An anonymous 40-something reader shared how her weight fluctuated in 1 day.

Time	Weight	Notes
7:15 a.m.	133.8 lb	Right before hopping in the shower
8:30 a.m.	137.5 lb	Wow, my clothes weigh 3.7 lb
9:15 a.m.	138.7 lb	Gained 1.2 lb from breakfast
10:30 a.m.	137.9 lb	Bathroom break, -0.8 lb
1:00 p.m.	135.8 lb	Lost 2.1 lb, thanks to a sweaty cardio workout
1:30 p.m.	137.4 lb	Up 1.6 lb from lunch
4:00 p.m.	138.6 lb	Gained 1.2 lb, probably from all the water I was drinking
5:30 p.m.	137.5 lb	Bathroom break, -1.1 lb
11:00 p.m.	140.8 lb	Yikes! Gained 3.3 lb—probably the pasta I ate and the wine!
11:30 p.m.	137.1 lb	Undressed—huh, gained 3.3 lb since this morning
7:15 a.m.	135.4 lb	Lost 1.7 lb while sleeping

12

Fast Track to a

FLAT BELLY

When you have diabetes, abdominal fat isn't doing you any favors. You can lose up to 4 pounds and 3 inches in 7 days with this incredibly effective, easy-to-follow routine.

Surprise! Good ol' crunches are one of the fastest ways to firm your midsection. (Hate crunches? Bear with us.) Thanks to 5 decades of research and nearly 90 studies, scientists have zeroed in on the best moves to flatten your belly. The secret is to really fatigue your abs, which is not an easy task, because they're used to working all day to keep you standing tall. But we created a routine that, when combined with regular cardio, does it in just four moves.

We know for sure because we had nearly a dozen women road test the program as part of our *Prevention* Fitness Lab.

"I couldn't believe the difference a few days made," says Gwen Hoover, 48, of Fogelsville, Pennsylvania, who whittled more than 2 inches off her middle, lost 14 percent of her belly fat, and dropped nearly 4 pounds in just 1 week! Even our slimmest testers saw impressive results. At 5 feet 6 inches and 125 pounds, Rachelle Vander Schaaf, 49, of Macungie, Pennsylvania, wasn't expecting to see a big change, but she shaved more than 3 inches off her belly—without dieting. You can, too! Start now and show off an all-around leaner belly—and fit back into your skinny jeans.

Program at a Glance

3 days a week. Do the four-move Slim Belly routine on 3 nonconsecutive days to tone your midsection.

5 days a week. Do 30 to 40 minutes of cardio, such as brisk walking, swimming, jogging, or bike riding, to burn off belly fat. You should be breathing hard but still able to talk in short sentences.

Every day. Watch your portions and fill up on whole grains, vegetables, fruits, lean protein, and healthy fats to maximize your results. Aim for 1,600 to 1,800 calories and spread them evenly throughout the day. To easily keep tabs on your eating, go to www.prevention.com/healthtracker.

Sample Workout Schedule

Here's what a typical week on the program should look like.

Day	Activity
Monday	Abs and cardio
Tuesday	Cardio
Wednesday	Rest
Thursday	Abs and cardio
Friday	Rest
Saturday	Abs and cardio
Sunday	Cardio

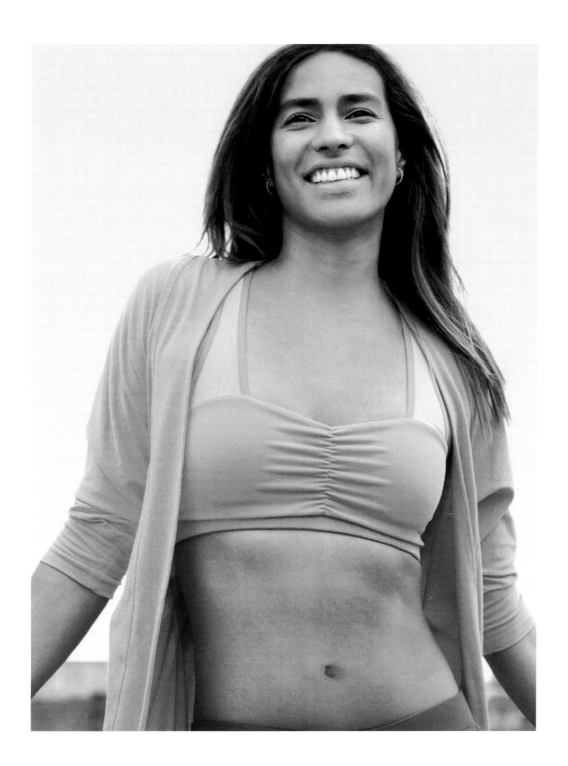

The Slim Belly Workout

Do 3 sets of each move, performing as many reps (1 second up, 1 second down) as possible until you feel a burning sensation in the muscles you're working or you can no longer maintain proper form. Rest for 15 seconds between sets. You'll likely be able to do more reps during earlier sets and exercises, and that's okay. After you can do 50 reps or hold a plank for 2 minutes for most sets, try the harder variations, change the order of the exercises, or do the moves after another type of workout.

THE EXPERT Tony Caterisano, PhD, exercise scientist and professor in the department of health sciences at Furman University, designed this workout.

50 YEARS OF FLAT ABS

Workouts to flatten belly bulge have changed plenty over the last half century, but each ab evolution brought us one step closer to the ultraeffective routine we're using today. Here's a look back at the most popular belly busters.

1960s/1970s: Old-School Sit-Up. It targets only the topmost belly muscle (the rectus abdominis), and your hip muscles do a lot of the lifting. Straight-leg versions are also particularly tough on the back.

1980s: The Crunch. When studies revealed that the first 30 percent of a sit-up engages abs the most, crunches became popular. But good form is key. Keep your feet off the floor and don't pull on your head.

1990s/2000s: Plank Pose. This Pilates move might work abs harder than crunches, but done alone it may not fully fatigue abs. Planks rely on smaller muscles that often tire more quickly.

Today: The Slim Belly Workout. It works! Researchers placed electrodes (like those used for EKGs) on the bellies of hundreds of people as they crunched, balanced, and twisted to find the most effective moves.

Hipless Crunch

This variation better targets abs by preventing hips and upper body from helping you lift. Prevention Fitness Lab testers averaged 25 reps per set.

> Lie on your back with your legs lifted and bent, your calves parallel with the floor, and your feet relaxed. Cross your arms over your chest with your hands on your shoulders. Contract your abdominal muscles and lift your head, shoulders, and upper back about 30 degrees off of the floor. Lower without touching your head to the floor. Exhale as you lift; inhale as you lower.

> Tips: Don't pull your chin toward your chest. Focus on your abs doing the work; imagine sliding your rib cage toward your hips.

> Stop when you start pulling or jerking up with your head, neck, or shoulders or if you can't keep your neck or shoulders relaxed.

> **Make it easier.** Rest your calves on a chair and extend your arms down at your sides.

> **Make it harder.** Extend your legs straight up.

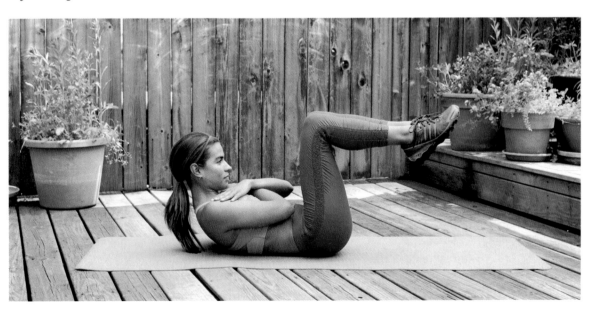

No-Hands Reverse Crunch

Instead of keeping your arms at your sides, where they can help your abs, anchor them overhead to activate more belly muscles. Prevention Fitness Lab testers averaged 21 reps per set.

> Lie faceup with your arms overhead and your hands grasping a heavy piece of furniture or railing. Raise your feet into the air with your legs bent. Contract your abs, press your back into the floor, and lift your hips off of the floor. Exhale as you lift; inhale as you lower.

> Tips: Feel the contraction in your abs, not in your back or legs. Tilt your pelvis. Think of lifting up instead of pulling your knees toward your chest.

> Stop when you can't lift your hips off of the floor without jerking or if your neck and shoulders are tense.

> **Make it easier.** Do the move with your arms down at your sides.

> **Make it harder.** Straighten your legs.

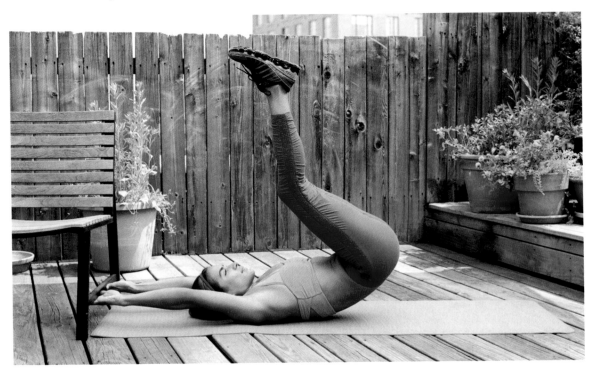

V Crunch

This exercise gets your upper and lower body moving simultaneously to recruit the maximum number of muscle fibers in your midsection. Prevention Fitness Lab testers averaged 11 reps per set.

> Balance on your tailbone with your legs bent, your feet off the floor, and your arms bent at your sides. Make sure that your back is straight and your chest is lifted. Lean back and extend your arms and legs, then pull back to the starting position.

> Tips: Your eyes gaze straight forward; keep your chin parallel with the floor. Don't let your back curve or your shoulders rise toward your ears.

> Stop when you can't keep your arms or legs up, if you can't keep your chest lifted, or if your back or neck starts to hurt.

> **Make it easier.** Grasp the sides of your thighs with your hands.

> **Make it harder.** Hold a 3- to 5-pound dumbbell in each hand.

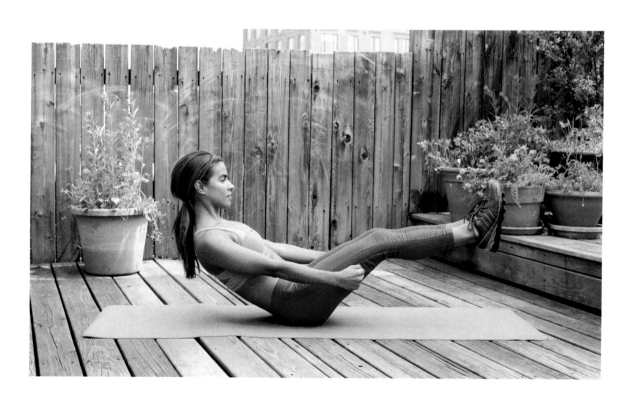

Side Plank

Static balancing moves like this one are challenging because your deepest abs work really hard to hold your core in midair. Do them after crunches to ensure complete fatigue and to firm abs from every angle. Prevention Fitness Lab testers averaged 19 seconds per side for each set.

> Lie on your right side, with your elbow beneath your shoulder, your feet stacked, and your left hand on your hip. Contract your abs to lift your hip and leg off the floor. Hold until fatigued, noting your time. Do 3 sets before switching sides.

> Tips: Keep your head, neck, torso, hips, and legs all in one straight line. Don't sink into your shoulder; press your elbow into the floor and lift your torso.

> Stop when your hip is sagging toward the floor, or if your neck, shoulder, or back hurts, or if you can't keep your body in line.

> **Make it easier.** Bend your legs and balance on your bottom knee and the side of your lower leg.

> **Make it harder.** Straighten your top arm toward the sky.

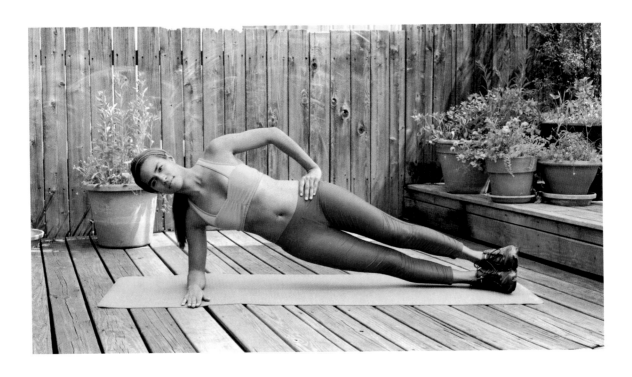

13

Are Your Bills Making

YOU FAT?

According to financial guru Suze Orman, climbing out of debt could help trim your waistline, too. They don't call it "belt tightening" for nothing.

Who would have suspected that getting a handle on your money woes could jump-start weight loss, too? It may sound far-fetched, but personal finance expert Suze Orman says she's seen it many times. In 2009, she famously predicted the winner of NBC's reality show *The Biggest Loser* based solely on his approach to finances. Although her initial pick in 2010 didn't take home the grand prize, he won the at-home portion of the show and actually lost the most weight overall (53 percent of body weight compared to the winner's 50 percent).

Although formal research in this area is slim (so to speak), a 2009 study from researchers at Harvard Medical School did confirm that stressing out over bills is associated with packing on pounds if you're overweight to start with.

"Finances were among the most consistent influences we saw [on stress-related weight gain]," says Jason Block, MD, lead author of the study and an instructor of medicine at Harvard Medical School. Orman's ideas, he says, make sense. But judge for yourself. Here's *Prevention*'s exclusive interview with Orman.

Prevention: How did you first make the connection between weight and problems with finances?

Orman: In 1999, when I was working on my book *The Courage to Be Rich*, there was a chapter called "For Love and Money," for which I was interviewing women in a relationship. I'm not sure why, but I started asking, "Are you overweight or underweight?" If they said "a little over," I'd ask how much over. It turned out that whenever they were hiding credit card debt from their husbands, there was a 2-pound weight gain for every $1,000 of hidden debt. So if they had $15,000 in hidden debt, they would be 30 pounds overweight. On my TV show, every time somebody was hiding debt—say, $10,000—I would do the math and ask, "Are you 20 pounds overweight?" They'd say, "Yeah, how did you know?" They thought I was psychic.

How do you account for this?

It's almost as if you're holding on to this shame, so you comfort yourself with food.

Have you found any research on this, or is it just your observation?

It's what I've found in more than 10 years of doing my books and *The Suze Orman Show*, with person after person calling in. But they're totally connected. If you're not balancing your checkbook and you don't know where your money is going, chances are you're not disciplined about what you put in your mouth either.

How did this play out when you were invited on *The Biggest Loser*?

I figured if my theory was correct, being good with money would lead to

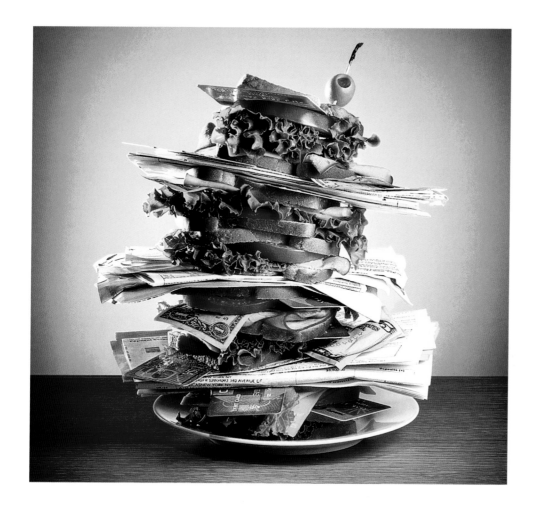

more weight loss. In season eight, Danny had the highest FICO score [a type of credit score], so I predicted he would win. And he did.

But Danny also had a lot of debt.

He had $45,000 in credit card debt, much of it from gambling—and he had hidden a lot of it from his wife. However, he got out of debt before becoming a contestant on the show. He went on to lose 239 pounds. When Danny came on my show after he won *The Biggest Loser,*

he said he couldn't have gotten rid of the weight without first getting rid of the debt. And he wouldn't have been able to keep the weight off without being debt free because it changed how he felt about himself.

Is developing discipline the key?

It's not discipline but a desire to be in control of your life. It's only when the pleasure of saving is greater than the pleasure of spending, or the pleasure of being fit and thin is greater than the

TRYING TO DOWNSIZE?

Whether you're reducing your debt or your waistline, the advice can be remarkably similar. We spoke with Catherine Williams, vice president of financial literacy for Money Management International, and Paula Ricke, a weight-loss specialist at the Mayo Clinic.

Be a "journalist." Write down every dollar you spend or calorie you eat in a journal (or spreadsheet or iPhone app). "Without it, you don't know your spending or eating patterns," says Williams. "You don't know how to attack the problem."

Devise a plan. Once you've figured out the patterns in your behavior, see where you can trim.

Make small, doable changes. Don't go for the quick fix. It took years to run up the debt, Williams says. You'll need time to pay it down. "People who fall for quick debt-resolution schemes often end up owing more money in the end." Sound like any crash diets you've ever been on?

Invoke the 24-hour (or 10-minute) rule. When the urge to splurge strikes, says Williams, wait for 24 hours before pulling out the credit card. Often the desire will pass. Of course, you can't wait a day for food. "But by waiting 10 minutes, you can often outlast a craving," says Ricke.

Anticipate lapses. They're normal. Ricke and Williams concur: "Just don't use them as excuses to give up."

pleasure of eating junk food, that you get it. You're saying, "I don't want that second piece of pie, or I don't want to buy those shoes, because ultimately it's not going to make me feel good."

You're filling an appetite in a different way.

Too many people eat and spend out of control because they're empty inside. They think they will fill up, but they never do. Or they're afraid. They think if they don't buy that item on sale now, it won't be there when they come back, or if they don't eat that dish, they won't be able to get it later. But those are the same shoes you put in your closet and never wear. And that pie sits unused in your body's fat closet.

But clearly there are exceptions. I know some gorgeous, slender women who are struggling with massive credit card debt.

In some cases, gorgeous women get into trouble financially because they want to look the part, with designer clothes and seriously expensive shoes, the greatest creams, and getting their hair and nails done. They're keeping up with the image.

What about the flip side—heavy women who are financial whizzes?

There are many factors besides debt that can get you into trouble with your weight. If it's not money, it's unhappy relationships or uncertainty about where you're going in life. But if you feel good about who you are, chances are you will be good with your finances and you should have what it takes to deal with your weight.

On some level, is this blaming the victim? Poverty is also a major predictor of obesity, since cheap food—sodas, chips, fast-food burgers, fries—tends to be unhealthy.

My original statement wasn't "if you don't have money." It was "if you have hidden credit card debt." I will be the first to say that if you have no money—and one in seven people in this country is on food stamps—you will be more likely to be overweight because of the choices that are available.

How would you characterize your own diet?

Fabulous, except that every so often I want a serious treat. In general, I eat no wheat, corn, or sugar. I try to stay away from meat. I eat only organic. I'm very disciplined. However, I'm about 20 pounds overweight because I hurt my back a year and a half ago and I can't exercise. I'm 59. When you get older, you have to exercise.

Are we going to see the "Suze Orman Diet"?

No, never. But will you hear me trying to connect being healthier and wealthier? Absolutely.

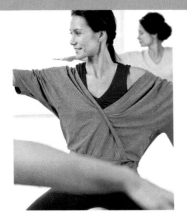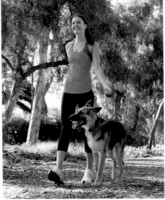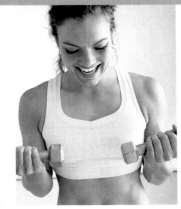

FITNESS
Medical Breakthroughs

When you have diabetes, it's important to exercise safely. Be sure to discuss it with your health-care practitioner and get her okay—particularly if you're over age 35; have had type 2 diabetes for more than 10 years; have heart disease or a strong family history of heart disease, high cholesterol, or high blood pressure; or have diabetes-related eye problems, nerve damage, foot injuries, or circulation problems. Your health-care practitioner might want you to take an exercise stress test to evaluate how healthy your heart is first.

MOTIVATE YOURSELF

You'll be more likely to work out if you focus on "how" to exercise instead of "why," found Texas Christian University researchers. One group of couch potatoes listed why cardio was good for them. The other group wrote down how they could do more, like "keep a pair of walking shoes in car" or "plan workouts the night before." After 2 months, the "how" group was exercising 25 minutes more per week. The strategies they came up with may have helped them overcome obstacles that can derail workouts, the researchers suspect.

Talk with Your Doctor

Before you begin an exercise program, it's a great idea to discuss the following exercise-related issues with your physician.

Foot care. One in four people with diabetes develops foot complications, thanks to reduced blood circulation and nerve damage that allow "little" problems like blisters to become major infections. Be sure to inspect your feet every day, looking for even tiny skin problems such as redness, chafing, blisters, sores, or cuts.

Ask your doctor what to look for, how to treat little problems, and when a foot problem deserves a trip to her office. You should also wash and dry your feet carefully every day, then apply a moisturizer made for people with diabetes. Ask your doctor for a recommendation. And ask how often you should have your feet examined by your doctor. Once a year is the general rule, but you may need more frequent checks as you become physically active.

Hydration. Hot-weather exercising could raise your risk for dehydration, especially if your blood sugar isn't well controlled. The reason: High blood sugar levels lead to more urination and to a reduced sense of thirst, so you end up with more fluid leaving your body and less coming in.

But the opposite is also true: Dehydration can cause your blood sugar level to rise. It's smart to sip 12 to 16 ounces of water before you begin exercising and another 4 ounces (that's $1/2$ cup) every 15 to 20 minutes while you're exercising. Ask your doctor how you can recognize signs of dehydration.

A medical alert bracelet. If you're exercising alone, a medical ID could save your life in the event of an emergency. Ask your doctor what it should say.

■ FIX DIABETES WITH YOGA

Yoga has a well-earned reputation as a surefire stress reducer (particularly when combined with meditation), and new studies show the simple stretching regimen can also help treat and prevent a number of other ailments, including diabetes. Unfortunately, less than 15 percent of women over age 35 say they do yoga frequently, according to the National Sporting Goods Association. Here, new research reveals four ways your health improves every time you strike a pose.

Yoga reverses metabolic syndrome. People at high risk for developing diabetes lowered their risk factors for the disease—including high BMI, blood pressure, insulin, and total and LDL cholesterol levels—after doing yoga for 3 months.

Yoga eases backaches. Chronic lower back pain sufferers had less pain and depression after practicing yoga twice a week for 6 months, according to *The Spine Journal*.

Yoga soothes asthma. After doing $2^1/_2$ hours of yoga a week for 10 weeks, asthma patients reported reduced symptoms, found the *American College of Sports Medicine*.

Yoga prevents mindless eating. Binge eaters who participated in a 10-week yoga therapy program reduced the number of bingeing episodes per week from five to an average of less than two, found the University of the Rockies.

"By teaching people how to be present, yoga helped participants develop

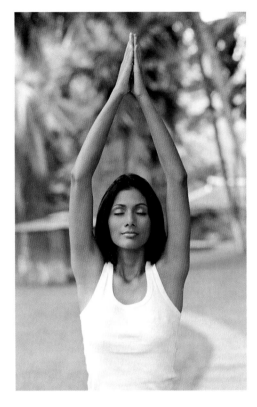

healthier strategies to deal with emotions that previously led to binges," says study author Debby Patz Clarke, PsyD.

Whatever your ailment, odds are you can help heal it with yoga.

■ SLOW DOWN TO REDUCE BLOOD SUGAR—AND MORE

The simple act of exercising—regardless of your weight or fitness level—can make you feel better about how you look, possibly a result of the release of feel-good hormones, finds a review of 57 studies on exercise and body image. Here's how.

A flat belly. Just two 40-minute workouts a week is enough to stop dangerous

The percentage increase in artery dilation among heart disease patients who did yoga for 6 weeks.

69

belly fat in its tracks, according to University of Alabama at Birmingham research. The waistlines of those who worked out less expanded an average of 3 inches. Exercise may lower levels of hormones such as cortisol that promote belly fat.

Healthy blood sugar. Walking 2 miles five times a week might be more effective at preventing diabetes than running nearly twice as much, report Duke University researchers. Because fat is the primary fuel for moderate exercise, walking might better improve the body's ability to release insulin and control blood sugar.

ERASE AGE WITH EXERCISE

Here's a snapshot of all the ways that staying fit can keep you healthy for years.

Better memory. Exercising at least three times a week at a moderate to high intensity can reduce odds of mental decline like dementia by 46 percent, according to a study of adults over age 55.

Stronger bones. Lifting weights twice a week can boost bone density and decrease falls by 40 percent, reports a study of 246 women ages 65 and older. Participants also stretched and did balance exercises 2 days a week.

Healthier body. Women who walk at a brisk pace at age 60 are up to 200 percent more likely to remain disease free at age 70, compared with casual walkers, found the Nurses' Health Study.

TAKE THE DOG

To burn up to 30 percent more calories, head out with a pup, say University of Missouri researchers. In a 12-week study, they found that dog walkers increased their speed by 28 percent (nearly a half mile an hour), while human walking partners went only 4 percent faster. Researchers suspect that the canines' enthusiasm encouraged faster tempos. When people paired up, they often talked each other out of going farther and even made excuses for skipping walks. No dog? Shelters always need walkers.

TAKE SIMPLE STEPS TO SLIM

Little moves, such as parking in the farthest spot, really do help you lose more weight, even if you work out regularly. When 34 women followed the same fitness plan for 8 weeks, some lost up to 7 pounds of body fat, while others gained as many as 5 pounds, found one study. The reason for this 12-pound difference: The biggest losers were active all day long—walking, climbing stairs, even fidgeting—while the gainers decreased their movements.

GET A 20-SOMETHING METABOLISM!

Want your college body back? According to new research conducted in London, lifting weights might restore muscle-building capability to the same level it was in your twenties, which is the key to a faster metabolism.

Researchers suspect that blood flow to

The percentage of dog owners who walk 30 minutes or more a day.

42

The number of extra calories you can burn daily by adding strength training to your routine.

105

muscles slows with age, so muscles get less of the nutrients that they need to repair and rebuild. When sedentary adults over age 45 did eight strength moves three times a week, blood flow increased, and they gained as much strength as younger lifters.

So grab a set of dumbbells and burn fat like a kid.

■ FLIP FOR FIRMER ARMS

For totally toned arms, flip your grip. Changing hand positions for dumbbell exercises targets different, often underutilized, muscles for allover firming, says exercise physiologist Pete McCall of the American Council on Exercise. Start biceps curls with palms facing back instead of forward. As you lift, they'll face away from you. Do triceps kickbacks with palms forward instead of in toward your body (lean forward with your arms bent 90 degrees, elbows by hips). Your palms will face down as your arms extend.

The Workout for Every Body—
WITH DIABETES

Whether you're just getting started or need a boost, you'll get the results you want with our customizable plans.

Some experts describe exercise as medicine without the pill, and for good reason. Name just about any chronic health problem, and exercise probably can help control it, if not reverse it.

Type 2 diabetes is a perfect example. Time and again, research has shown that regular physical activity helps lower blood sugar because the body uses insulin more efficiently. In fact, people with type 2 diabetes who are taking medication are often able to reduce their dosages once they begin a fitness routine. Likewise, those who aren't taking medication may not need it quite so soon, if at all.

For exercise to have any benefit, of course, we need to actually do it. And there's the rub. Eating, like breathing, is essential to our survival, and so we make a point of doing it on a fairly regular schedule. Exercise... well, let's be honest. When our days get hectic, as they do more often than not, our workouts are the first things to go. We tell ourselves with all sincerity that we'll pick up where we left off tomorrow, or the next day, or the day after that. Pretty soon we've been away from it for so long that we ask ourselves, Why bother?

Why, indeed. Because even though we can live without exercise we risk our long-term health when we do.

For the next few weeks, we want you to think of exercise not as an expense, but as an investment. Yes, you're setting aside time that you could be using for something else. But you're buying a stake in your future, in years of good health and independence.

We also encourage you to consider physical activity not as time spent away from life, but in the thick of it. Motion is life. Moving your body can be fun. And watching it become slimmer, stronger, and healthier is incredibly rewarding and motivating.

Science-Based Routine, Real-World Results

As you might imagine, the science of fitness is growing by leaps and bounds, with researchers regularly announcing fantastic new discoveries about the health effects of various forms of physical activity. One particularly impressive study, the Diabetes Aerobic and Resistance Exercise (DARE) study, was conducted at the University of Ottawa in Canada.

The research team behind DARE determined that both aerobic exercise (also called cardiovascular exercise, or cardio for short) and strength training (that is, lifting weights) can help people with type 2 diabetes lower their blood sugar. What's more, the combination of cardio and strength training controls blood sugar significantly better than either activity alone.

It isn't news that cardio and strength

training individually help prevent or manage type 2 diabetes. Previous studies, for example, have found that aerobic exercise—the kind that elevates the heart rate for a sustained period—helps lower blood sugar and LDL cholesterol while raising HDL cholesterol (the good kind).

But the DARE study—published in 2007 in the *Annals of Internal Medicine*—was the first to assess the collective effects of both forms of activity on blood sugar.

For this study, the researchers divided 251 people with type 2 diabetes into four groups. Three of the groups worked out

GOT DIABETES? BE SMART ABOUT WORKING OUT

There's no doubt that exercise can be a real asset in managing diabetes. It stabilizes blood sugar not only by helping cells use insulin more effectively, but also by burning off excess body fat, which further improves insulin response.

If you have diabetes, you need to be somewhat choosy about how much exercise you get and what kinds. Some activities might not be right for you, especially if you're experiencing complications such as heart disease, kidney disease, or eye or foot problems.

Your doctor can start you on the right path by reviewing your workout ideas with you and suggesting adjustments based on your health status and fitness level. The following pointers can help, too.

If you have diabetes-related eye problems. Too-heavy weights can increase the pressure in the blood vessels of your eyes. Ask your doctor how much you can safely lift.

If nerve damage has made your feet numb. You might want to choose an aerobic activity other than walking, such as bicycling or swimming. Discuss the options with your doctor. If he gives you the all clear to walk, be sure to wear shoes that fit. Check your feet for any sores, bumps, or redness after every workout.

If you take a diabetes medication that can cause low blood sugar. You might need to adjust your dosage before your workout, or eat a snack if your blood sugar is below 100. Ask your doctor what's best for you.

After your workout. Check your blood sugar. If it's below 70, have one of the following immediately:

3 or 4 glucose tablets or 1 serving of glucose gel (15 grams carbohydrate)

½ cup fruit juice

5 or 6 pieces of hard candy

1 tablespoon of sugar or honey

After 15 minutes, check your blood sugar again. If it's still low, go back for another "dose." Repeat until your blood sugar is 70 or higher.

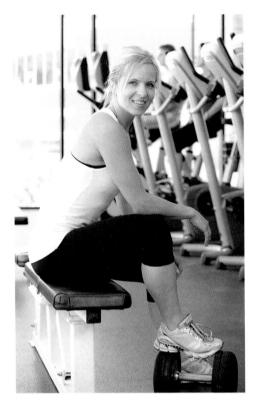

aerobic exercise and strength training, fared even better: Their collective A1c value fell an additional 0.46 percent over the aerobic-only group and 0.59 percent over the strength-training-only group. Compared to controls, the combination exercisers had a nearly 1 percent lower A1c reading.

This might seem like a modest change, but it comes with huge benefits. Consider this: A 1-point drop in A1c—which, you'll remember, reflects average blood sugar over several months—is associated with a 15 to 20 percent reduction in risk of heart attack and stroke and a 37 percent reduction in diabetes-related complications, such as kidney, eye, and limb damage.

The Workout for Every Body

If there's one absolute truth about exercise, it's that it is never too late to start. At 45, Sandra Wright weighed 242 pounds and began with just 5 minutes a day on a $5 garage sale stationary bike. In a year, she pedaled off 100 pounds. That is what's thrilling about exercise. Once you take the first step, you'll get results fast. In fact, new or lapsed exercisers could boost aerobic capacity by 25 percent after just 8 weeks, says Cedric Bryant, PhD, chief science officer for the American Council on Exercise. That means you'll have more energy, and all types of activities will feel easier.

We recruited experts who specialize in

for 45 minutes 3 days a week; the fourth, "control" group did no exercise at all. Group 1 walked on treadmills or rode exercise bikes, both of which qualify as aerobic exercise. Group 2 used weight machines, a form of strength training. Group 3 did both.

Over the course of 6 months, the researchers saw improvements in the blood sugar readings of all the exercise groups. Compared with the control group, Group 1 shaved 0.51 percent off their collective hemoglobin A1c value, while Group 2 showed a reduction of 0.38 percent. Group 3, which did both

helping women of all sizes and ages overcome exercise barriers. Their personalized plans ease you into working out, no matter what your starting level. Bonus: We made sure to keep it fun—a key to motivation.

HOW TO PERSONALIZE YOUR ROUTINE

Pick a plan. If you're new to exercise, haven't worked out in 6 months or more, or need to ease into a program because of health issues, follow Plan 1.

If you stopped exercising within the past 6 months, use Plan 2. (See page 134.)

If you exercise but need a push to stay motivated or break through a plateau, go with Plan 3. (See page 134.)

Choose your fun! Each plan integrates Cardio Intervals (pick any activity you like—walking, jogging, or elliptical), Feel-Good Firming moves (see page 137) to tone your body and increase energy, and Fun Activities (see page 135) to broaden your idea of exercise and make it something you look forward to.

Plan 1: Get Started

Begin with short bouts of exercise and lengthen your workouts gradually. You'll burn more calories without overtaxing your muscles and joints or feeling overwhelmed.

WEEK 1

Monday/Thursday. Cardio Intervals: Two 10-minute cycles

Tuesday/Friday. Feel-Good Firming move #1 (see page 137)

Wednesday/Saturday. Rest

Sunday. Fun Activity: 15–20 minutes (see page 135)

WEEK 2

Monday/Thursday. Cardio Intervals: Two 15-minute cycles

Tuesday/Friday. Feel-Good Firming moves #1 and #2

Wednesday/Saturday. Rest

Sunday. Fun Activity: 20–30 minutes

WEEK 3

Monday/Thursday. Cardio Intervals: One 30-minute or two 15-minute cycles

Tuesday/Friday. Feel-Good Firming moves #1, #2, and #3

Wednesday. Rest

Saturday. Rest or Fun Activity

Sunday. Fun Activity: 30 minutes or more

WEEK 4

Monday/Thursday. Cardio Intervals: One 40-minute or two shorter cycles

Tuesday/Friday. Full Feel-Good Firming routine

THE EXPERTS Fabio Comana, exercise physiologist, personal trainer, and fitness educator for the American Council on Exercise, designed the cardio routines. Rochelle Rice, president of the In Fitness & In Health studio in New York City and author of *Real Fitness for Real Women*, designed the strength workout.

Wednesday/Saturday. Rest or Fun Activity

Sunday. Fun Activity: 30 minutes or more

NEXT STEPS

When the Week 4 workouts feel manageable and you're ready for a new challenge, move on to Plan 2.

Plan 2: Back Up to Speed

Your past fitness prowess pays off, as your body will adapt quickly when you start working out again. "Long-term exercise (a year or more) creates lasting changes in the heart and muscles, even if you stop being active," says William Kraus, MD, an exercise physiologist at Duke University School of Medicine.

WEEK 1

Monday/Wednesday/Thursday/Saturday. 30-minute Cardio Interval or Fun Activity

Tuesday/Friday. Feel-Good Firming routine (see page 137)

Sunday. Rest or Fun Activity

WEEK 2

Monday/Thursday. Cardio Intervals: 5 minutes at an easy pace, then alternate 3 minutes at a difficult-to-talk pace with 6 minutes at a catch-your-breath pace. Do two 3-minute/6-minute cycles. Cool down with 5 minutes at an easy pace (total workout time: 28 minutes)

Tuesday/Friday. Feel-Good Firming routine

Wednesday/Saturday. 30-minute Cardio Interval or Fun Activity

Sunday. Rest or Fun Activity

WEEK 3

Monday/Thursday. Cardio Intervals. Same as Week 2, but do three 4-minute/6-minute cycles (total workout time: 40 minutes)

Tuesday/Friday. Feel-Good Firming routine

Wednesday/Saturday. 30-minute Cardio Interval or Fun Activity

Sunday. Rest or Fun Activity

WEEK 4

Monday/Thursday. Cardio Intervals. Same as Week 3, but do four 4-minute/6-minute cycles (total workout time: 50 minutes)

Tuesday/Friday. Feel-Good Firming routine

Wednesday/Saturday. 30-minute Cardio Interval or Fun Activity

Sunday. Rest or Fun Activity

NEXT STEPS

When the Week 4 workouts feel manageable and you're ready for a new challenge, move on to Plan 3.

Plan 3: Take It to the Next Level

"By increasing from two or three workouts a week to five or six and adding intervals to my walks, I lost 20 pounds in 4 months and lowered my blood pressure and cholesterol," says Angel Smedley, 40.

WEEK 1

Monday/Wednesday/Friday. Cardio Intervals: 5 minutes at an easy pace, then alternate 3 minutes at a vigorous, can-barely-talk pace with 6 minutes at a catch-your-breath pace. Do the 3-minute/6-minute cycle four times. Cool down with 5 minutes at an easy pace (total workout time: 46 minutes).

Tuesday/Thursday. Feel-Good Firming routine (see page 137)

Saturday. 30-minute Cardio Interval or Fun Activity

Sunday. Rest or Fun Activity

WEEK 2

Monday/Wednesday/Friday. Cardio Intervals: Same as Week 1, but do five 3-minute/5-minute cycles (total workout time: 50 minutes)

Tuesday/Thursday. Feel-Good Firming routine

Saturday. 30-minute Cardio Interval or Fun Activity

Sunday. Rest or Fun Activity

WEEK 3

Monday/Wednesday/Friday. Cardio Intervals: Same as Week 2, but do six 3-minute/4-minute cycles (total workout time: 52 minutes)

Tuesday/Thursday. Feel-Good Firming routine two times

Saturday. 30-minute Cardio Interval or Fun Activity

Sunday. Rest or Fun Activity

WEEK 4

Monday/Wednesday/Friday. Cardio Intervals: Same as Week 3, but do seven 3-minute/3-minute cycles (total workout time: 52 minutes)

Tuesday/Thursday. Feel-Good Firming routine two times

Saturday. 30-minute Cardio Interval or Fun Activity

Sunday. Rest or Fun Activity

NEXT STEPS

Continue the Week 4 schedule, sampling different interval lengths and recovering for the same time (such as 2 minutes hard/2 minutes easy or 6 minutes hard/6 minutes easy).

Fun Activities!

Finding enjoyable ways to move your body—beyond cardio machines and pedometers—really helps make exercise a pleasurable habit. Here are six we swear by, with tips on how to get going.

BIKING

Wind in your hair, the open road ahead—turns out the childhood favorite is a top-notch calorie burner, melting about 540 an hour.

Beginner's block. A literal pain in the butt (or knees).

Overcome it. The number one mistake: a seat that's too low, according to Christine Mattheis, associate editor of *Prevention*'s sister publication *Bicycling*. "When your leg is down in the 6 o'clock position, it should be extended with only a slight bend." Sore backside? Opt for a padded seat or padded bike shorts, but not both.

More info. Find expert advice, gear reviews, local routes, and two-wheeling inspiration at www.bicycling.com.

DANCING

If *Dancing with the Stars* has you tapping your feet, try ballroom or swing with a partner, or tap, jazz, or line dancing if you're going solo.

Beginner's block. Following the choreography.

Overcome it. Start with a beginner's class, and take it one step at a time. Usually the instructor will build on a basic step, mixing it up and adding arm movements. Stick with the basic until you're ready to add on.

More info. Check for classes at your local YMCA or community center, or at www.meetup.org.

YOGA

There's no better way to stretch away stress, loosen tight muscles, and make you feel like a new person.

Beginner's block. Poor balance.

Overcome it. "Picking a spot to focus on helped me stop wobbling," says Kathyanne White, 59, adding that she also learned to laugh at herself when she did topple.

More info. Go to www.yogaalliance.org to find credentialed instructors in your area, or try free daily podcast classes at www.yogatoday.com.

SWIMMING

If you're overweight, have joint problems, or just want a change of pace, exercising in water will make you feel lighter and more graceful. The built-in resistance also gives you a total-body workout that's easy on your joints.

Beginner's block. Bathing suit confidence.

Overcome it. Check out a company specializing in larger sizes, such as Junonia (junonia.com), for a suit that boasts wide straps, a neckline that doesn't scoop water, and a "magic vent" that keeps skirted styles from bubbling up.

More info. Find everything from local pools to lap-swimming etiquette to workouts at www.usmastersswimming.org.

TEAM SPORTS

A recent study of sedentary British women who attended soccer practices twice a week found that the fitness benefits—like increased fat burn, strength, and lung capacity—trumped those of traditional workouts like running.

Beginner's block. Thinking you don't have time.

Overcome it. Contrary to the common assumption that do-anytime workouts are best, the soccer players in the study showed up for more workouts than the runners did, finding that set practice times (plus the camaraderie of teammates) made workouts easier to fit in.

More info. Find local teams and leagues for more than 20 sports and activities at www.active.com.

KICKBOXING

Throwing punches and jabs is a proven stress buster that burns about 680 calories an hour.

Beginner's block. Feeling like you have two left feet (or fists).

Overcome it. "Go slow until you master the form," says Jessica Smith, personal trainer and star of the *10 Minute Solution: KnockOut Body!* DVD. "If you can't keep up, perform every other punch with the instructor," she suggests, "and exhale when you punch or kick. It gives you more power and helps you remember to breathe!"

More info. Go to www.collagevideo.com for DVDs to try at home.

Feel-Good Firming!

Get strong, be confident.

Strength-training boosts your energy, so you'll want to move every chance you get. Refer to your personal plan for when and how to do this routine. Do 10 to 15 reps of each exercise. When using dumbbells, choose a weight that tires you out by the last rep (about 3 to 8 pounds to start). If you can't do at least 8 reps, you need a lighter weight. Once you can easily do 15 reps of an exercise, increase the amount.

Bent Rows

> Sit with your feet flat, with a dumbbell in each hand, your arms at your sides, and your palms facing in. Bend forward at your hips, keeping your back straight. Pull the dumbbells straight up toward your chest, rotating your arms so your palms face behind you and your elbows are bent out to the sides. Slowly lower.

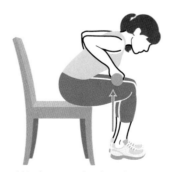

Works upper back and arms

Rocker Squat

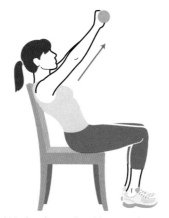

Works butt and thighs

> Sit on the edge of a chair, with your feet hip-width apart, your knees directly over your ankles, and your arms bent in front of you. Rock forward, shifting your weight onto your feet and lifting your hips about 6 inches off the chair. Pause; slowly sit back down. For a challenge, hold dumbbells.

Recline Press

Works chest, shoulders, and arms

> Sit on the edge of the chair, with your shoulders resting on the chair back (use a pillow if needed). Hold weights by your shoulders, with your elbows pointing out, and your palms away from you. Straighten your arms, pushing the weights up and forward on a diagonal. Slowly lower back to the start.

Raised Plank

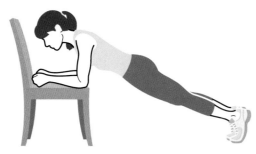

Works shoulders, arms, chest, back, and abs

> Place your forearms on the chair seat (pushed against a wall if needed), and walk your feet back until your body forms a straight line from your head to your heels. Hold for 15 to 30 seconds, taking a break if needed. For a challenge, place your forearms on the floor.

15

Fun: The New WORKOUT

Here are great ideas to get moving, pump up energy, and make fitness part of your everyday life.

Who says exercise has to be work? Just head outdoors and start having fun! Here are wonderful ways to make fitness fun.

Remember when you were a kid, and the activities you did outside—biking, swimming, playing tag—never felt like work, but pure pleasure? You can easily recapture that feeling again as a grown-up. All it takes is a little outdoor exploration.

Even traditional exercise feels easier and more enjoyable when you do it outside, and your energy levels will soar. New activities also naturally shape and slim your body as you use new muscles to maximize calorie burn. You'll have so much fun you won't even notice that you're working out.

The beauty of exercising outdoors is that the sky, literally, is the limit. Here, our 13 favorite activities with smart ideas on how to get started. Consider this your chance to get happy, healthy, and strong while having fun with family or friends, or capturing some much-needed "me" time.

Bike Riding: Nostalgia Galore

The fastest route to feeling like a kid again is to hop on a bike, even if it's been years since your last ride. Along the way, you'll burn more than 500 calories an hour pedaling at a relatively moderate pace, while sculpting your legs and butt without stressing your knees.

Yes, you can! Whether you rent, borrow, or pull an old bike out of the garage, two key moves will keep you comfortable: Inflate your tires and check your seat height.

"The softer your tires, the harder it will be to ride," says John Howard, author of *Mastering Cycling.* And to avoid a sore rear, make sure your leg is extended with only a slight bend when it's in the 6 o'clock position.

Try before you buy! RentaBikeNow.com lists rentals in hundreds of cities and offers roadside assistance and free bad weather cancellations. If you want to avoid cars, go to www.traillink.com to find bike paths in your area.

Trail Running: A Scenic De-Stressor

When you're out on the trail running, it's more about appreciating what's around you than worrying about how fast you're going. In fact, it's often better to take some walking breaks, especially on hilly or uneven terrain. But you'll burn about 30 percent more calories than when hiking (about 600 an hour).

Yes, you can! Lots of people avoid running because it hurts their joints, but dirt trails have softer impact. Just choose a shorter route than normal.

"Running on a hilly trail will take longer than on the road," says Nancy Hobbs,

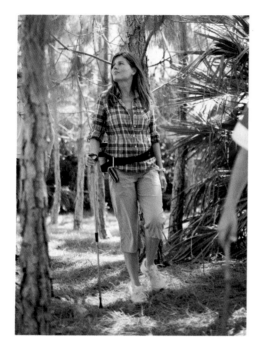

with directions or know how to use a compass. Just go to www.geocaching.com to choose a cache. Then plug the coordinates into a handheld GPS or a cell phone with built-in GPS. Start with a 1/1 rated cache—which means it's not too hard to find and on relatively easy terrain—and look for any location hints on the Web site.

Try before you buy! If you don't want to invest in a GPS (they cost about $100 and up), some libraries and parks rent devices for the day.

In-Line Skating: The Joy of Speed

Runners and walkers will be excited to cover more ground, burn more calories—upward of 800 an hour—and sculpt the underused muscles in their inner thighs and hips. You can do it anywhere there's pavement: Sneak in a quick lunchtime workout or have a "chat and roll" with a pal.

Yes, you can! Even beginners will have a blast because this low-impact activity is easy to pick up. Practice good form while stationary on grass or carpet: knees bent so you can't see your toes, hands in front of you, and pelvis tucked, says Liz Miller, author of *Get Rolling: The Beginner's Guide to In-Line Skating.* To brake: Slide right foot forward at least 10 inches, then lift toe. (If you're left-handed, switch the brake to your left skate for better balance.)

Try it! Visit www.getrolling.com for

executive director of the American Trail Running Association.

Try it! Regular running shoes will get you started. Invest in trail running shoes if you head out more than once a week. For trails and more beginner tips, go to www.trailrunner.com.

Geocaching: A Hiking Treasure Hunt

The thrill of searching for one of a million treasures or caches (typically, small plastic boxes holding trinkets and a log book) turns a walk in the woods into your own *Survivor* adventure. As you explore your surroundings, you'll burn about 400 calories an hour.

Yes, you can! You don't have to be good

The percentage of people who experience an increase in self-esteem after a nature hike.

90

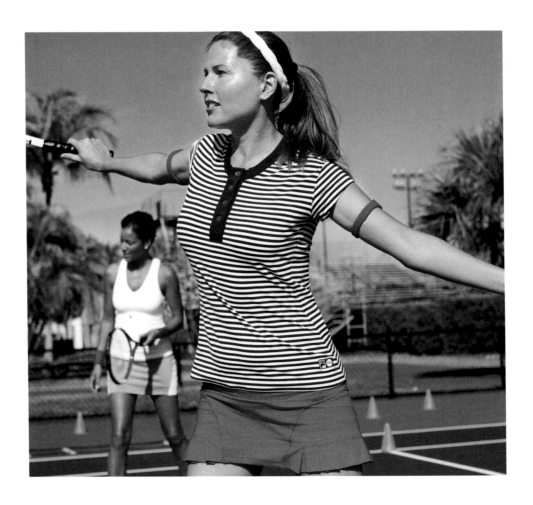

loads of beginner-friendly tips and free instructional videos.

Boot Camp: The Perfect Girlfriend Workout

Time to drop your to-do list and let someone else be in charge for an hour. Get back to basics—such as jumping jacks, running, squats, and push-ups—with lots of fresh air to keep you energized from start to finish. Whether your group uses resistance bands and light weights or relies on rocks, logs, and anything else Mother Nature might offer, you can expect to burn about 450 calories an hour while toning your muscles from head to toe.

Yes, you can! You don't have to be able to do full push-ups or scale walls to join. Most instructors work with all fitness levels and provide modifications for difficult moves, while other participants often offer encouragement and help.

Try it! Search for a boot camp class near you at outdoor-fitness-bootcamp. meetup.com.

BACKYARD FUN!

Want to inject some healthy energy into your family bonding time? Pry everyone away from their BlackBerrys, laptops, and video games with these time-tested games. They are ranked 1–4, from the easiest to the most challenging.

Badminton = 4. There's no keeping score. No net? Just volley to see how long you can keep the shuttlecock in the air. Count the hits and aim for more each time. Costs $15 and up for rackets and birdies.

Frisbee = 2. No catching required. Pick a target and play Bull's-Eye: Take turns throwing the Frisbee to see whose shot lands the closest, and mark the spots if you're playing with just one Frisbee. Costs $8 to $20 for a Frisbee.

Shooting hoops = 3. Dribbling is optional! Challenge everyone to a game of Around the World. Shoot from five or seven spots in an arc around the basket. (Younger players can stand closer.) Every time you sink one, move to the next spot. The first one to finish wins. Costs $10 and up for a ball.

Bocce ball = 1. Easier than bowling: Just toss the pallino, a small ball, onto the grass. Then try to get your balls as close as possible. To keep the game fair, have the most skilled players throw with their nondominant hand. Costs $20 to $40 for a set.

Hopscotch = 4. Challenge both kids and adults and race to see who can hop through the pattern the fastest. (Search "hopscotch diagram" online if you need to see what it looks like.) To really test your stability, throw two stones, one at the start and one at the end, to hop over two squares each time. Or use a coin because it's harder to pick up than a stone. Costs $2 to $5 for a box of chalk to draw the diagram.

Cardio Tennis: Recess for Adults

Channel your inner Serena by learning tennis basics, from baseline sprints to forehand and backhand shots. Take your stress out on the ball while sculpting your legs, arms, chest, shoulders, and core. It's all set to music and done in a group, for a truly energizing experience that burns around 350 to 500 calories an hour.

Yes, you can! Don't let the name fool you. You don't even have to know how to play tennis!

"The class isn't concerned with where or how you hit the ball—or if you miss it altogether—because no one is keeping score," says Michele Krause, national manager of the Cardio Tennis program.

Try it! You can find a Cardio Tennis class near you at cardiotennis.com.

Fly-Fishing: A Moving Meditation

The rhythm of casting the line and feeling the water flowing past you makes fly-fishing extremely meditative, and adds

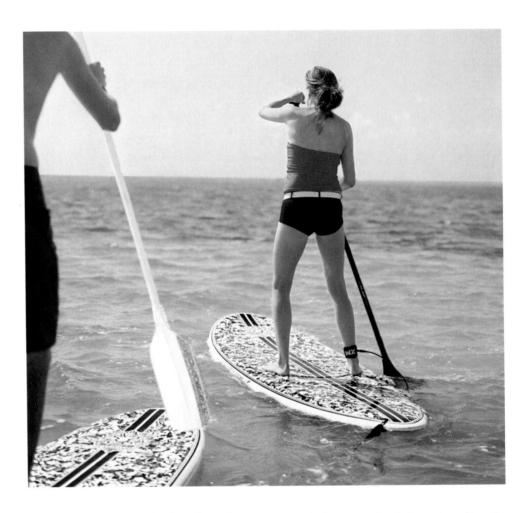

up to a surprisingly high calorie burn (more than 400 an hour, about the same as a brisk walk uphill).

Yes, you can! You don't have to travel to Montana or Alaska to get a taste of fly-fishing. While you do need the basic gear (rod, reel, waders for cold water, flies, and a license), some of the 250-plus fly-fishing clubs nationwide might loan out equipment. And getting the hang of casting requires no more coordination than swinging a golf club or a tennis racket.

Try before you buy! Search online to find a fly-fishing school near you. Or go to the Federation of Fly Fishers Web site at fedflyfishers.org to locate a club that offers clinics.

Stand-Up Paddling: A Tranquil Ab Workout

Anyone who's ever honeymooned in Hawaii has seen stand-up fans navigating ocean waves with their paddles.

Stop Watching and Start Moving

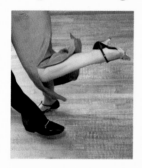

Rainy or cold day? Love *Dancing with the Stars?* Then get motivated to find your groove. You don't need a pro to show you how to dance off up to 500 calories an hour, whether you're a natural born boogier or a shy, hug-the-sidelines type. Regardless of the dancing style you choose (disco, salsa, ballet), shaking your booty to the beat lifts your spirits even more than other forms of exercise do. And it's easy to get started, no rhythm required. Here's how to find the venue that's right for you.

Couples. Go to a local salsa night or sign up for a lesson.

No partner? Organized events often attract solo dancers. To find lessons, check with local studios or go to accessdance.com.

Two left feet. Get down in your living room with a DVD. You will feel less self-conscious and can rewind to master any tricky steps. We like *Dance Your Ass Off: The Workout* ($16, collagevideo.com).

Former clubber. Dance Dance Party Party hosts all-women events at more convenient times (like early evening) in 12 cities. Find an event at dancedancepartyparty.com or throw your own.

Choreography-phobe. Try Nia, a movement class done barefoot to music. An instructor gives some sequences to get you started, then you do your own thing. Find a class at www.nianow.com.

Rhythm queen. You'll love Zumba, an easy-to-follow class set to Latin beats. Go to www.zumba.com for classes or DVDs.

The average weight loss after 6 to 9 hour-long dance workouts over 3 weeks, according to *Applied Human Science*.

7 pounds

Today the sport—a combination of surfing and kayaking—is popping up on rivers, lakes, and ocean inlets throughout the country as a low-key way to spend time on the water while going at your own speed. Paddle fast and you'll get an aerobic challenge (and burn about 400 calories an hour), or go slow and enjoy the Zen vibe.

Yes, you can! It's easier than it looks! Stand-up boards are larger than surfboards and designed to be very stable. It's rare for even beginners to fall, but if you do, it's all part of the fun (and a good way to cool off!).

Try before you buy! Many surf shops and outdoor sports centers rent boards; search "stand-up paddle rentals" and your location. Check out an instructional video on YouTube; search "SUP: How To."

GET OUT OF THE GYM

. . . and into the great outdoors! Walking hilly terrain scorches about 500 calories an hour and seriously shapes your legs and butt, and, according to studies, walking in nature can significantly improve your mood. Start with comfortable, broken-in hiking shoes. (We like Keen Obsidian WP, about $125; keenfootwear.com.) Here's the best gear to stay dry, energized, and firmly on the trail.

Rain layer. Showers can sneak up. This waterproof and windproof jacket folds to the size of an apple. (Marmot Crystalline jacket, $130; marmot.com)

A map. Not an app! Weather- and tear-proof maps withstand all conditions, and unlike your smartphone, they're never out of range. (Nat Geo Trails Illustrated maps, $12; natgeomaps.com)

30+ SPF sunscreen. Rays are stronger at higher elevations. As you remove layers, apply a sweat-resistant formula. (Coppertone Sport Ultra Sweatproof Sunscreen, $10; drugstores)

A thirst-quenching backpack. The best models—like the Gregory Maya ($99; gregorypacks.com for retailers)—hold a hydration reservoir (CamelBak; various sizes, $25 to $30; camelbak.com) for hands-free sipping. External pockets are handy, and a waist belt lightens the load on shoulders. Visit www.prevention.com/packs for more.

Amber shades. Even in fall and winter, sunlight might seem dimmer, but the UV rays are still damaging. An amber tint provides crisper vision. (Suncloud Daybreak, $49; suncloudoptics.com)

Trail mix. Snack on Bear Naked Trail Mix in Pecan Apple Flax ($3; bearnaked.com) for an energizing mix of protein, carbs, and fat. For full-day hikes, also bring fresh fruit and a sandwich.

Walking poles. Lightweight poles can ease knee pressure during descents by up to 25 percent. They also boost calorie burn and aid balance. (Leki Cressida Aergon Trekking Poles, $119; leki.com)

16

The Wonder of

WALKING

Pick your goal and discover a fun new way to achieve it.

Weight. Fatigue. Trouble zones.

Whether you want to melt fat, boost energy, lift mood, or just be a bit more toned in a few important places, we have the workouts for you. They've all been road tested by *Prevention* readers and are ready to deliver fast results. Pick your goal and change your body—and your life.

Your Goal: Flip Your Fat-Burning Switch!

You could shrink a size (or more) this month by adding high-intensity walks to your routine. You'll burn more fat during and after your workouts. There are options to fit everyone's needs, including a 10-minute routine for busy days and an indoor option for rainy weather.

For best results, do at least 20 minutes of high-intensity walking (any combination of the workouts in this section or any of the hill or stair routines on page 158; the longer walks will slim you down faster) on 3 nonconsecutive days a week. On alternate days, do moderate-intensity activity for about 30 minutes per session.

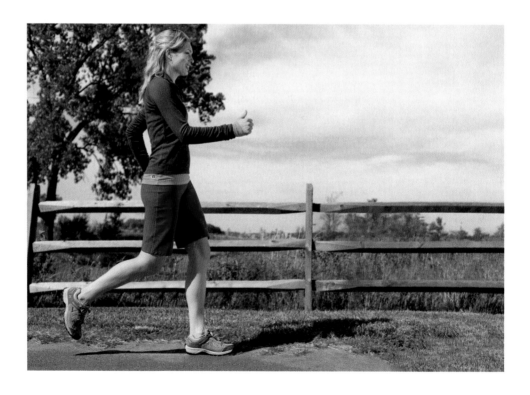

TREADMILL SLIMMER

30 minutes

Treadmills are the perfect excuse buster. There's no need to worry about weather, traffic, or darkness. Seeing your speed increase as you become more fit is also a huge motivator. Try the routine below from Lee Scott, creator of the DVD *Simple Secrets for a Great Walking Workout,* to blast more than 150 calories in half an hour. (All calorie burns are based on a 150-pound person and will vary depending on weight, walking speed, and workout duration.)

Start at a comfortable speed. Increase 0.6 mph from there for Phase 1 speed intervals. For each subsequent phase, increase your speed intervals by 0.2 mph.

DROP-IT-FAST SPRINT

25 to 30 minutes

The quicker you walk, the farther you can go, and the more pounds you'll melt off. Here's a fun routine that burns as many as 175 calories.

THE WORKOUT

After warming up for 5 minutes, walk as fast as you can for 10 minutes. Note how far you went. Then turn around and walk back at a brisk pace, slowing your speed to cool down as you get closer to your

Time	Activity	Speed
0:00–4:59	Warm-up	3.4 mph
5:00–10:59	Phase 1 (repeat intervals below for 6 minutes)	
	60-second speed interval	4.0 mph
	60-second recovery interval	3.4 mph
11:00–15:59	Phase 2 (repeat for 5 minutes)	
	40-second speed interval	4.2 mph
	20-second recovery interval	3.4 mph
16:00–20:59	Phase 3 (repeat for 5 minutes)	
	30-second speed interval	4.4 mph
	30-second recovery interval	3.4 mph
21:00–25:59	Phase 4 (repeat for 5 minutes)	
	20-second speed interval	4.6 mph
	40-second recovery interval	3.4 mph
26:00–30:00	Cool-down	3.4 mph

starting point. Each time you do this workout, aim to walk faster and go farther than your initial turnaround point.

MEGACALORIE BURNER

60+ minutes

This is perfect for the weekend! Hour-plus workouts can crank up your postexercise calorie burn nearly fivefold compared with a 30-minute walk. That's on top of the nearly 350 calories you'll melt during your walk. This can also get you in shape to take on a bigger goal, such as a half marathon (13.1 miles) or a multi-day fund-raising walk.

It's also a social way to slim down: Plan your route so you meet up with friends, and walk with each other for part of your route.

"Meeting someone along the way helped keep me from getting bored," says *Prevention* reader Kim Kline of Jefferson City, Missouri.

SUPER FAT BLAST

10 minutes

This one is a great time-saver. (See chart below.) Crank up the intensity with metabolism-revving bursts of high-impact activities. You'll burn nearly 70 percent more calories than if you walked at a steady pace.

BELLY-BUSTING WALK

10+ minutes

High-intensity workouts like the ones in this section can shrink five times more belly fat than moderate-intensity workouts. To zero in on shaping your abs, use these toning tips during any walk.

Focus on drawing your abs in toward your

Time	Activity
0:00–2:59	Warm-up, easy to moderate pace
3:00–3:59	Brisk walk
4:00–4:29	Jog
4:30–5:29	Fast walk
5:30–5:59	Jumping jacks in place
6:00–6:59	Fast walk
7:00–7:29	Side jumps, feet together, in place
7:30–8:29	Fast walk
8:30–8:59	Jog
9:00–10:00	Cool-down, easy pace

spine. Try to maintain the contraction throughout your walk, but don't hold your breath.

Imagine that your legs extend up above your navel. As one leg swings forward and back, that hip should follow. This slight hip swivel causes your lower torso to rotate, activating more ab muscles to tone your midsection faster.

Your Goal: More Energy and a Brighter Mood

Even a 10-minute stroll can instantly recharge your energy by increasing circulation. Go for 30 minutes and you could get a whopping 85 percent energy boost, research shows. And to really wake up your body and brain, try the following stimulating walks that get your mind and senses working, too. The good feeling may last up to 12 hours!

Any time you need a quick pick-me-up, try one of these routines. These workouts can also help if your goal is to lose weight or firm up.

HAPPINESS WALK
10+ minutes

Revitalize your mind and body with an easy walk of any length that includes the following stress-busting techniques from Carolyn Scott Kortge, author of *Healing Walks for Hard Times.* Says *Prevention* reader Lisa DiMarzio of Ware, Massachusetts: "When I tried it after a tense meeting, I felt calm almost immediately

Phone a Friend

Working out à deux can make a tough routine feel easier. A University of Oxford study found that exercisers tolerated discomfort better when working out in a group, compared with going it alone. Researchers believe partner workouts may heighten levels of hormones such as endorphins that boost mood and block pain signals.

Take-home tip. Grab a friend or two when you want a kick-butt workout. The camaraderie will make it easier for you to push yourself and get faster results than exercising alone.

instead of reliving the event that made me stressed."

Step 1: Focus on your feet. Feel the firm ground beneath you as each foot rolls from heel to toe. Try to hold awareness of your steps for 2 to 3 minutes.

Step 2: Turn your attention to breathing. Lift your torso to stand upright and increase lung space. As you inhale, imagine you are drawing in renewed energy. Exhale tiredness and pain. Let fresh life flow into your lungs and your cells.

Step 3: Mentally talk to yourself. Thinking "fresh air in, stale air out" as you breathe can help you maintain focus.

GEAR UP FOR YOUR WALKS

Everyone needs good shoes and socks for exercising, but it's even more important if you have diabetes. Worn-out shoes can contribute to foot, knee, and back pain. If you have diabetes, the added risk for circulation and nerve problems means it's also important to protect against blisters, sores, and chafing. Follow these steps for the perfect footwear.

Find a knowledgeable salesperson. Unlike mass-market retailers, specialty stores often employ trained shoe fitters who will ask you about your walking habits and watch you walk. This information will improve your chances of getting the right shoe for your feet.

Get your feet measured. Your size can change over time, and footwear that's too small or too narrow can set you up for an array of problems. Make sure you have a thumb's width of room in front of the end of your big toe while you're standing rather than sitting. Make sure the width of the shoes is comfortable, too.

Replace your shoes every 300 to 500 miles. That's about every 5 to 8 months if you're walking about 3 miles 5 days a week. By the time a sneaker looks trashed on the outside, the inside support and cushioning are long gone.

Invest in "wicking" socks. Look for synthetic fabrics that wick moisture away, keeping your feet dry and making them less prone to blisters. Since some are thick and others are thin, wear your walking socks when you try shoes on because they can affect the fit. If you get the proper fit and fabric, you probably don't need to invest in specially marketed diabetic socks.

BRAINPOWER BOOSTER
Under 20 minutes

This walk targets inner thighs. Changing the direction you walk—forward, backward, or sideways—keeps your mind alert, turns up your calorie burn, and activates some often-underused muscles, such as your inner and outer thighs. This routine is best done on a school track (most are $\frac{1}{4}$ mile around).

THE WORKOUT
Lap 1. Start at the beginning of the curved part of the track. Walk as you normally would to warm up for a full lap.

Lap 2. Turn sideways so your right foot is in front. Sidestep or shuffle around the curved part of the track.

Walk backward on the straight section.

Sidestep through the next curve with your left foot in front.

Walk forward on the straight section.

Lap 3. Repeat Lap 2, walking sideways, backward, sideways, and forward.

Lap 4. Walk forward, slowing your pace to cool down.

This is a 1-mile walk if you use a $\frac{1}{4}$-mile track. You can do more laps to extend it or work up to doing half or even full laps of each type of walking.

HEAD FOR THE TREES

5+ minutes

A dose of nature can boost your mood and energize you in just 5 minutes. If you exercise in a natural setting and go longer (a lunchtime stroll in a park or an all-day hike in the mountains), you can improve your memory and attention 20 percent more than you can by walking in an urban environment. That's because there are fewer distractions and it's more relaxing. To find off-road walking routes in your area, go to www.trails.com.

Your Goal: Firm Your Arms, Butt, and Thighs

By adding some toning moves or techniques to your routine, you can turn walks into total-body workouts and shape your legs and butt even faster.

Aim to target each body area two or three times a week. For example, do the Sculpt All Over (see page 158) once or twice a week, and do a lower-body and an upper-body routine (or two) on alternate days. Don't work the same muscle groups on back-to-back days. For speedier firming, do walking routines from other sections on in-between days to melt flab and show off your sexy muscles.

DOUBLE-DUTY TONER

10+ minutes

Use a pair of walking poles ($90 and up). Research shows they can boost calorie burn by up to 46 percent and get your arms and core involved for allover firming. The poles also reduce impact on your joints. Go to www.nordicwalkingna.com for more information.

Walk Off 8 Pounds This Year

All you have to do is make one simple change! Just swap your watch for a pedometer. Studies show that this simple change can encourage you to walk an extra 2,000 steps a day. To push your number—and your weight loss—even higher, make it a game.

Here's how: Compete with your family to see who can get more steps by the end of the day. The winner picks what's for dinner.

Walk in place anytime you're standing still—say, when talking on the phone or waiting for the microwave—and see how many more steps you rack up.

Do shopping laps. If you can't break the habit of parking as close as possible to the grocery store, take a lap as soon as you get inside.

TREADMILL BOOTY BLAST

25 minutes

No outdoor hills to give your glutes a workout? Here's a fun treadmill routine from Tracey Staehle, a Connecticut-based trainer and creator of the DVD *Walking Strong*. Reports *Prevention* reader Carrie Pasquale of Petal, Mississippi: "I could really feel it in my butt." You can do the full 25-minute routine or

Activity	Time	Speed (mph)	Percentage Incline
Warm-up	0:00–4:59	2.5	0
		Increase speed 0.2 mph and incline 1 percent each minute	
Gradual ascent	5:00–9:59	3.3	5
		Maintain speed but increase incline 1 percent each minute	
Rolling hills	10:00–10:59	3.4	5
	11:00–11:59	3.5	5
	12:00–12:29	3.7	7
	12:30–12:59	3.7	5
	13:00–13:29	3.8	8
	13:30–13:59	3.8	5
	14:00–14:29	4.0	10
	14:30–14:59	3.5	5
Steep climb	15:00–19:59	2.6	10
		Maintain incline as you increase speed 0.3 mph each minute	
Cool-down	20:00–25:00	3.4	4
		Decrease speed 0.2 mph and incline 1 percent each minute	

ACCESSORIZE!

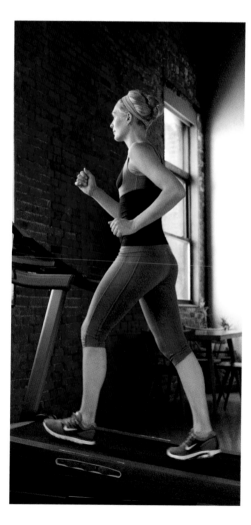

just one or two of the 5-minute hill climbs for a shorter session.

ARM SHAPER

20 minutes

This is a great workout for your lunch break. Grab an exercise band and do these moves while you walk to firm your upper body.

THE WORKOUT

Start with 4 minutes of easy walking. Then pick up your pace to a moderate intensity and do the first exercise on pages 156–157 for 25 reps. When you're finished, drape the band around your neck and speed up to a brisk pace, like you're in a hurry, for 2 minutes. Repeat the 25-rep toning/2-minute brisk-walking intervals until you've done all the exercises. Cool down with 4 minutes of easy walking. You can make the moves harder by placing your hands closer together so you're using less band, or easier by separating your hands for more slack.

Shoulder Shaper

> Loop the band around your back. Hold each side with your palms up, your elbows bent in at your waist, and your forearms angled out to the sides (A). Keeping your shoulders down and back, press your hands up and away from your body to about shoulder height (B). Slowly lower to the starting position.

Chest Circle

> With the band around your back, extend your arms in front of you, crossing your wrists (A). Circle your arms out to the sides (B), bend your elbows, and bring your hands in to your chest. Repeat, crossing your opposite arm on top.

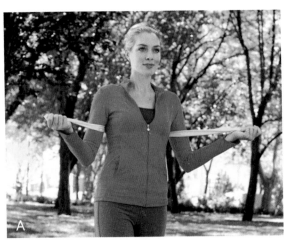

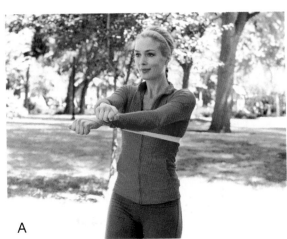

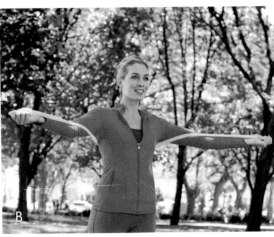

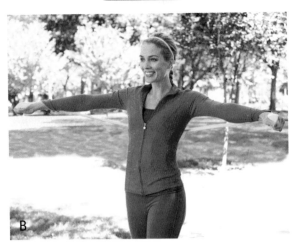

Back Pulldown

› Hold the band wide overhead (A). Lower your arms, keeping your elbows bent slightly (B), and pull the band down behind your head. Slowly return to the starting position.

Triceps Toner

› Hold the band at shoulder height in front of you, with your hands wide and your elbows bent 90 degrees (A). Keeping your upper arms still, straighten your arms and press your hands out to the sides (B). Slowly return to the starting position.

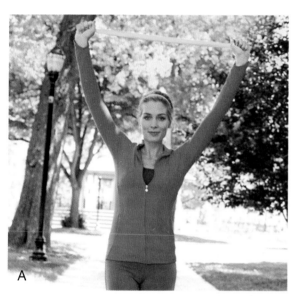

A

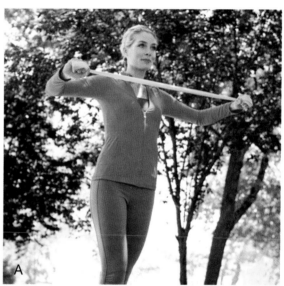

A

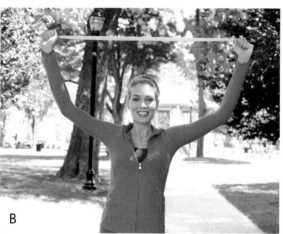

B

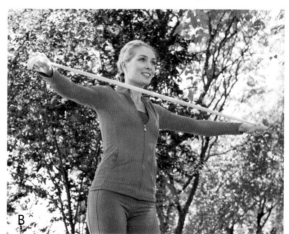

B

BUTT FIRMER

16+ minutes

Walking uphill activates 25 percent more muscle fibers for faster firming than strolling on flat terrain. For best results, find a hill that takes 2 to $2\frac{1}{2}$ minutes to climb and try the following workout from Judy Heller, a certified personal trainer and master racewalker in Portland, Oregon.

THE WORKOUT

Warm up at an easy pace for 5 to 10 minutes. Then walk up and down the hill; follow with 2 minutes of brisk walking on a level surface. Repeat the hill and level walk to increase your workout length. Finish with 5 minutes of easy walking to cool down.

SCULPT ALL OVER

25 to 40 minutes

During this workout, you'll intersperse strength moves as you walk, for cardio plus toning. Using this lottery approach from Lee Scott to pick your exercises will prevent boredom.

THE WORKOUT

Write at least nine strength moves on pieces of paper. Vary exercises to hit all major muscle groups, such as walking lunges, bench push-ups, triceps dips, planks, and power jumps. Drop them in a jar and draw three out before a walk. Warm up at an easy pace for 3 to 5 minutes, then walk briskly for 5 to 10 minutes. Stop and do one of the strength moves. Repeat the brisk walking (5 to 10 minutes), followed by the next strength move. Repeat once more to complete the final move. Cool down for 5 minutes at an easy pace.

INDOOR LEG TONER

5 minutes

This is an easy home routine. Do this quick workout anywhere there are stairs to double your calorie burn.

1. Walk up and down one flight normally.

2. Slowly walk up sideways, crossing your bottom foot over your top. Keep your head up. Walk down normally. Repeat, facing the opposite direction.

3. Step up on the first stair, then down, starting with your right foot (right up, left up, right down, left down) 10 times. Repeat, starting with your left foot.

4. Climb the stairs two steps at a time; come down quickly using each step.

5. Run up; walk down normally.

6. Repeat numbers 4 and 5 another four times.

7. At the bottom, place your right foot on the first or second step, bend your knees, and lower into a lunge. Keep your right knee directly over your ankle as you do so. Push off with your right foot to return to the starting position. Repeat with your left leg. Alternate legs for 20 lunges total.

8. Walk up and down normally one time.

THE EXPERT Michele Stanten, author of *Walk Off Weight*, designed several of these workouts.

Bicycling for a

BETTER YOU

Prevention came to the rescue of Jackson, Mississippi, one of the diabetes capitals in the nation, by getting residents to hop on bikes. Now you can, too!

Type 2 diabetes has reached epidemic proportions in this country. Even teenagers, who were not considered at risk for the disease in prior generations, are being diagnosed. The culprit? Growing rates of obesity—or, as some doctors now refer to the intertwined problems, "diabesity." According to the American Diabetes Association, as many as 25.8 million Americans have some form of the disease and another 79 million are at risk—together, nearly one-third of the country.

Diabetes has been called a silent killer because it won't make you feel ill immediately. But the accumulated damage from high blood sugar levels can eventually lead to heart disease, nerve damage, amputations, kidney failure, and diabetic retinopathy (the leading cause of blindness in adults over age 19). Since 1987, the death rate from the disease has climbed by 45 percent, according to the American Diabetes Association.

But you can vastly reduce your risks just by tweaking your diet and boosting activity levels. Shockingly, most doctors don't make a serious effort to discuss these options with their patients, in large part because they don't think people will make the needed changes when they can just pop a pill. But at *Prevention* we've seen how readers can and do change their lifestyles and are much happier. Here, we show you how. Just follow our diet guidelines, and grab a bike.

Follow a Disease-Busting Diet

Eating in a diabetes-friendly way can help you cover all the nutritional bases, while getting out of the diabetes danger zone or avoiding it in the first place. Here are simple guidelines to follow.

Check your calories. Aim to eat around 1,400 to 1,600 calories each day.

Put fat cells on a diet. Though it's not totally clear why, vitamin D, omega-3 fatty acids, and calcium work together to help torch fat and boost your metabolic rate, so you'll want to eat plenty of these. Aside from the obvious sources, you can find surprising amounts of calcium in tofu, cooked collards and spinach, oatmeal, and canned white beans. Both vitamin D and omega-3s are found in salmon and sardines, and omega-3s are also in walnuts and ground flaxseed.

Make friends with fiber. When Finnish researchers tracked 4,316 men and women for over 10 years, they found that those who ate the most fiber were 61 percent less likely to develop type 2 diabetes. Fiber-rich foods (fruits, vegetables, beans, and whole grains) deliver more nutrients for fewer calories. And because they have more volume, they keep you feeling fuller longer.

Eat more often. That's right. Having some healthy food every 3 hours will help

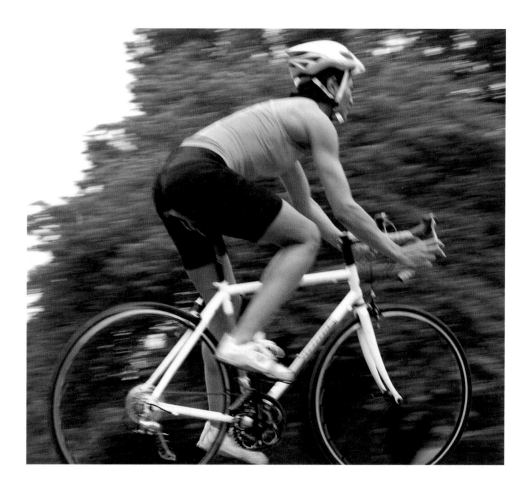

prevent the munchies and keep your blood sugar levels stable. Aim for three meals and two snacks a day. And whatever you do, don't skip breakfast.

Learn delicious diabetes-fighting recipes. At the end of this book, you'll find 100 diabetes-friendly recipes. They're delicious and nutritious.

Pedal Off the Pounds

Hour for hour, biking beats walking for calorie burn. A 150-pound rider taking a leisurely spin around the neighborhood uses 272 calories in 60 minutes—even taking coasting into account—versus 224 for a moderate hour's walk at 3 mph. Ramp your cycling up to a doable 13 mph and the total goes up to around 544 calories. You'd have to do an hour of speedwalking at 5 mph to blast that many calories. But when you compare the energy used to cover a set distance—say, from home to the office—you'll probably work off more by walking because you'll spend longer doing it.

(continued on page 164)

ACROSS THE FINISH LINE

Twelve lucky contestants qualified for the *Prevention* and *Bicycling* BikeTown program in Jackson, Mississippi. They took home free Jamis Commuter 1 bikes, along with copies of *The Diabetes DTOUR Diet* and *The Diabetes DTOUR Diet Cookbook*. Three months later, the winners were delighted with the improvements in their lives. Here are a few of our all-stars.

LISA RATZLAFF

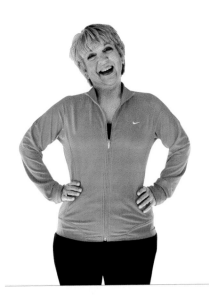

Ratzlaff is a 54-year-old stay-at-home mom who lost 11 pounds and $3\frac{1}{2}$ inches off her waist.

"I didn't feel good and had no energy. But I had this vision of riding a bike as I used to as a little girl, with the wind in my hair," Lisa says.

"I've gone from being prediabetic to having normal, healthy blood sugar levels. I've lost two dress sizes, and I will actually wear sleeveless shirts. I used to be a typical Southern cook, with lots of sauces and fried food. When I ate vegetables, they were flavored with bacon grease. Now I cook the DTOUR recipes and share them with my best friend. I have more energy, more drive, more optimism."

TESHEBA EPPS

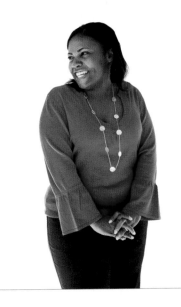

Epps is a 31-year-old nursing student who lost 10 pounds and 4 inches off her waist.

"I just wanted my own bike. I've always had to share or borrow. I felt that having a bike would change my world because I could ride with my two boys and become fit while spending time with them." Though she was not prediabetic, a family history of diabetes worried her.

"I feel so free when I ride, and it relieves my stress," Epps says. "[The bike and the diet] have both been a blessing from God."

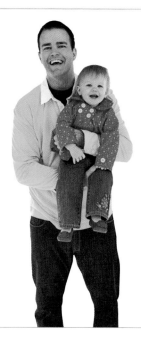

BRAD BUMGARNER

Brad is a 37-year-old mechanical engineer who lost 16 pounds and 3 inches off his waist.

After losing a diabetic grandmother and learning that his mother had been diagnosed with the disease, Brad feared he was heading toward diabetes himself. He wanted to be around to see his two young daughters grow up.

He's lost weight, feels better, and is out of the prediabetic zone, having brought his blood sugar levels down by one-third. His wife, Katie, told him that getting involved in the program was the best thing he'd ever done for the family. "It was the best compliment she's given me in five years of marriage," he says.

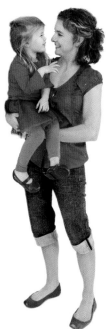

KATIE BUMGARNER

Katie is a 30-year-old realtor who lost 8 pounds and 4 inches off her waist.

Katie volunteered for the program to support her husband, Brad. But she also thought that having a bike would help her make up for the exercise she wasn't getting since giving birth to two girls, now 2 and 3. "No driving to the gym, just hop on my bike and go," she says.

"Our family has had fun getting fit. We'll ride to the duck pond or to the fountains, where my girls can play. We get exercise, and we can do it as a family."

Shopping for a bike can be as simple or as complicated as you let it be. For the best fits, our advice is to head to your local bike shop (as opposed to a big box store). They will have the expertise to help fit you, answer all your questions, and send you on your way. Here's what you need to know to get rolling.

THE RIDE

Consider a hybrid (bike, that is). If you're just starting out, you'll probably want to choose one of the commuter bikes, or hybrids, as they're also called. These models are a cross between the ultralight road bikes that are used for racing and the much heavier mountain bikes. Hybrids let you sit upright, with straight-across handlebars, comfortable saddles, and flat pedals (as opposed to the clipless pedals on racing bikes). Some models we like include the Jamis Commuter 1, the Breezer Uptown 8, and the Raleigh Detour Deluxe. Expect to spend anywhere from $365 for the Jamis to $879 for the Breezer.

Make sure the bike "fits." One of the great things about cycling is that it burns off a lot of calories with minimal impact on the joints. But it also involves a highly repetitive motion—cycling—so even small imperfections in the bike's fit will quickly become obvious. Most bike shops will help you choose a bike that's the right size for you: not too big, not too small, but in the Goldilocks zone—just right. But before buying, take your bike for a test spin to make sure. A good bike shop will let you.

Saddle up. Once you have the right size bike, you'll want the shop to adjust the seat. If it's too high, your hips will rock from side to side. If it's too low, you may feel pain in front of your knees. In some cases, you may want to swap out the seat for one that fits your booty better. A company called Specialized has an in-shop system that measures the distance between your sit bones, then uses that to select the ideal padded seat for you.

Get a grip. Commuter bikes come with straight-across or slightly curved handlebars to enable you to sit upright. They shouldn't be too much of a reach, which is another reason why getting a bike with the right fit is so important. Some riders buy special padded grips or wrap the handlebars with leather bar tape, which has a comfortable feel and absorbs sweat.

THE GEAR

Of course, you'll want some gear, too, and there are plenty of ways to indulge. But two items should be at the top of your wish list.

A helmet. This is your one absolute essential (other than the bike). A good option for beginners is the Giro Skyla Women's Helmet. It costs only about $40 but delivers just as much protection as more expensive models. (They all have to meet the same safety standards.) Just be sure to wear your helmet down over your forehead, so you can see the front of it when you look up. Otherwise, your head won't be fully protected in a headfirst crash. And pull the strap tight, so the helmet won't slip. There should be only a finger or two's worth of space between your chin and the strap.

Padded bike pants. They'll make the ride more comfortable, and believe us, your butt will thank you. Specialized Women's BG Comp Shorts ($90) are great for beginning bikers because they fit more like comfortable shorts than ultratight racing pants, but they have the same "chamois" padding. (Note: You're not supposed to wear underwear with them. Part of the point is to avoid extra seams rubbing and chafing against your skin. If you feel embarrassed wearing tight pants, pull baggy shorts or a short skirt on over them.)

The extras. Bike shops are full of cool stuff, including ventilated jerseys, sunglasses that change tint when you coast from the glaring sun into a tree-shaded alley, cages for your water bottle, tire pumps, lights that attach to the bike or your clothes, padded gloves, bike locks, and bike racks for your car. But you don't need to spring for these extras at this stage. You already have the essentials. With your bike, helmet, and pants, you're on a roll!

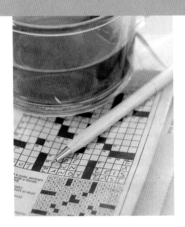 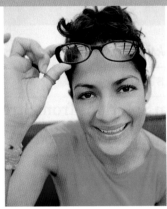 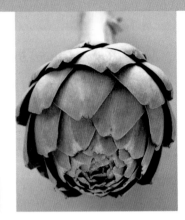

MIND-BODY
Medical Breakthroughs

Diabetes can cause many complications, including mental health ones. In people who have diabetes, the fight-or-flight response does not work well. Insulin is not always able to let the extra energy into the cells, so glucose piles up in the blood. As a result, long-term stress can cause long-term high blood glucose levels. To make matters worse, people under stress might not take good care of themselves. If you have diabetes, it's especially critical to adopt a healthy mental attitude and take good care of your mental health.

DON'T WORRY, EAT HAPPY

Thirty percent. That's the drop in your risk of depression if you eat a Mediterranean diet rich in produce, whole grains, healthy oils, and nuts. Researchers say essential nutrients in these foods help brain cells bind to serotonin, which is a mood-boosting neurotransmitter.

BOOST YOUR BRAINPOWER

A healthy lifestyle means a brighter mind. Recent studies reveal small tweaks to stay even sharper.

If you already get plenty of cardio…

Upgrade. Start lifting weights. The cognitive function of older people who strength trained once or twice a week improved nearly 12 percent, compared with that of women who followed a simple stretching and toning routine. The challenge of learning and mastering different moves can improve brain health.

If you already sleep on a big decision…

Upgrade. Fuel up on food, then decide. An empty stomach can make you more impulsive, found a University of South Dakota study. When you have enough calories, you can focus on the outcome of a tough choice instead of immediate needs, like food for survival.

If you already do the Sunday crossword…

Upgrade. Read, rest, and recall better. When New York University researchers looked at brain activity of study participants after they performed a memory test and then rested, the scientists observed increased activity in the areas linked to memory consolidation. "The brain replays images during rest, so you're more likely to remember them," says researcher Lila Davachi, PhD.

MUNCH THESE MEMORY BOOSTERS

Here's good news for adults who have trouble recalling words and names: A diet rich in luteolin, an antioxidant in certain vegetables and herbs, might help reduce brain drain, according to new research by the University of Illinois at Urbana-Champaign. Luteolin regulates immune cells in the brain called microglia. As we age, these cells begin overproducing inflammatory chemicals that cause forgetfulness, says study author Rod Johnson, PhD. Here are the top four sources:

Green bell pepper (1 medium): 5.9 milligrams

Artichoke (1 medium): 2.9 milligrams

Blueberries, frozen (1 cup): 2.8 milligrams

Hot green chile pepper (1 raw): 1.8 milligrams

KEEP SHARP WITH SPECS

Talk about rose-colored glasses! A recent University of Michigan study found that people with better vision (including those who wore corrective contacts or glasses) were 63 percent less likely to develop Alzheimer's disease over an $8\frac{1}{2}$-year period than those with poor eyesight who

The percentage of people who haven't been to an eye doctor in 5 years.

35

didn't fix it. Some vision problems and dementia may share the same underlying causes. Also, people who don't see well tend to avoid brain-boosting habits such as exercise, reading, and socializing.

■ AVOID SCARY STRESS

Stress is a national epidemic, but experts say the real worry is its wicked stepsister, burnout. The main difference? Stress makes you feel frazzled and overwhelmed, but burnout leaves you flattened and unmotivated. It's especially destructive: A recent Finnish study suggests that chronic burnout can be deadly, as it may cause depression and heart disease. Here's how to prevent or recover from it.

Reduce daily stressors. Unrelenting pressure plays a huge role in burnout onset, says psychologist Jeanne Segal, PhD, cofounder of helpguide.org. Zap stress in the moment with 10 minutes of exercise, such as a lap around the office. Also crucial: restorative habits, such as downtime away from work.

Volunteer with a mentoring program such as Big Brothers Big Sisters. Feeling under-appreciated is one trigger of burnout. Coaching others is shown to increase self-satisfaction, says California psychologist Shoshana Bennett, PhD.

Spread your wings at work. Burnout is especially linked to workplace woes, including feeling unchallenged. Lend new meaning to your daily grind: Take on a new project outside your comfort zone or sign up for continuing education classes to expand your skills.

■ STAY SLIM, STAY SHARP

If your scale registers a healthy weight, your mind is likely youthful, too. In a recent UCLA study, overweight people had 4 percent less brain tissue than normal-weight adults—the equivalent of their minds aging 8 years. One possible cause is a high-calorie or high-fat diet, which clogs arteries in the brain, restricts blood flow, and causes cells to shrink.

Stress BUSTERS!

Yes, diabetes is stressful. But everything you think you know about beating that stress is wrong. Read on for six smart new strategies to start now.

I f deep breaths, weekly yoga classes, and venting to your friends aren't helping you relax, you have plenty of company, and it's not your fault. New studies show that these supposedly tried-and-true anxiety busters are often just . . . well, a bust. Read on for the surprising truth about what really helps—and what doesn't—when it comes to relieving chronically fried nerves.

Yesterday's Wisdom:
Never Go to Bed Angry

Today's smart strategy: Just get some sleep already!

When you're mid-dustup and about to wring your husband's neck, the last thing you feel like doing is curling up in bed beside him. But deep down, many of us worry that going to bed angry just tempts fate. So we bargain, cajole, and then fight some more in an effort to resolve the dispute, thinking all will be well by the morning if we can just reach a resolution.

The fact is, forcing a discussion by bedtime can actually make things worse, says Andrea K. Wittenborn, PhD, an assistant professor in the marriage and family therapy program at Virginia Polytechnic Institute and State University. When you're upset, a part of the brain called the amygdala cues the fight-or-flight response, limiting your ability to have a calm, rational discussion. So it's a good idea to hold off on any showdown until you cool off.

"Taking a time-out or even a night off is critical, because once you've activated the fight-or-flight system, you can't simply tell it to turn off," says Ronald Potter-Efron, PhD, author of *Rage: A Step-by-Step Guide to Overcoming Explosive Anger.* "If you're already angry or frustrated, you become emotionally flooded and unable to think clearly."

Plus, sleep is a powerful antidote to stress, says Russell Rosenberg, PhD, director of the Atlanta Sleep Medicine Clinic and vice chairman of the National Sleep Foundation. Instead, agree to call a truce until morning, and make sure to actually talk things out the next day. "Completely dropping issues that really bug you can be damaging to your relationship and contribute to increased stress," warns Dr. Wittenborn.

Yesterday's Wisdom:
Control Your Temper

Today's smart strategy: Throw a tantrum now and then.

From the time we're little girls and boys, we're taught to control our tempers, and as adults—especially women—we still believe that venting anger is unhealthy (not to mention unladylike). In fact, the opposite now appears to be true. According to a study published in *Biological Psychiatry*

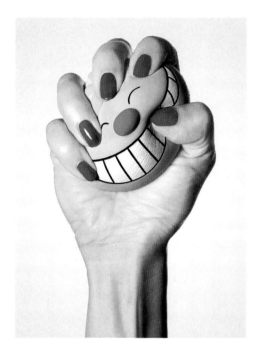

Today's smart strategy: Cuddle up with your pet.

Hanging out with loved ones has long been touted as an instant mood booster, but according to new scientific evidence, when it comes to managing stress, the calming effects of spending time with a furry friend trump those obtained by hanging out with friends and family.

"Having your pet, whether a cat or a dog, with you during a stressful event turns out to be more soothing than a best friend or a spouse," says James J. Blascovich, PhD, a professor of psychology at the University of California, Santa Barbara.

Dr. Blascovich and colleagues asked volunteers to perform difficult math problems while in the company of their spouse, a friend, or their pet. Using heart rate and blood pressure as measures of stress, the researchers found that people strained the least and performed the best when in the company of their cat or dog. While spending time with a friend or spouse can be a great way to relax, sidle up to your pet when the pressure's on.

Yesterday's Wisdom: Express Your Feelings

Today's smart strategy: Keep them to yourself.

In our tell-all, Oprah-fied culture, we've

that looked at the effect of facial expressions of emotions—such as fear and indignation—on our stress responses, displaying your anger might actually cause your brain to release less cortisol, which is the stress hormone associated with obesity, bone loss, and heart disease. And while experts know that chronic anger contributes to hypertension and coronary disease, they've also found that expressing irritation in response to a short-term and unfair frustration, such as being cut off in traffic, can actually dampen the nasty effects of stress. That's because anger confers feelings of control, counteracting the helplessness and frustration we often feel in response to perceived insults and injustices, says lead study author Jennifer Lerner, PhD.

(continued on page 176)

DE-STRESSING DESIGN

You spend such a significant portion of your life in your home. Why not make it into a low-stress haven? The choices you make can result in enhanced mood, less stress, and better sleep. To turn your space into a healing haven, follow these easy room-by-room tips.

ENTRYWAY

Create a feel-good focal point. The first thing you see when you enter your home should be something you love, whether that's a piece of art, a vase of flowers, or a special souvenir, says Stephanie Roberts, author of *Fast Feng Shui: 9 Simple Principles for Transforming Your Life by Energizing Your Home.* "A beautiful first impression helps you relax from the get-go."

Organize daily debris. If you see old newspapers on the floor and bags of Goodwill donations waiting to be dropped off, you're going to think obligation, not relaxation.

"Piles of stuff at your entryway send the message that there's more mess and chaos inside, and who wants to walk into that?" Roberts says. "Have a designated place for every item that enters and exits your house," recommends Paige Rien, an interior designer in New Jersey who appears on HGTV's *Hidden Potential.* She suggests placing a couple of chic containers near the front door, one for outgoing items and one for incoming things.

LIVING ROOM

Create space. "Our anxiety builds in small spaces if there's too much stuff," says Rien. To reduce the clutter and make the room feel larger, ask yourself if you really need all those end tables or picture frames, and cut anything deemed nonessential. Consider painting a table or bookshelf the same color (or a similar one) as the wall it's up against, so it "disappears" into it. Painting walls white or a light color will also make a smaller room feel more spacious.

Light up locations, not whole rooms. "Bright overhead light can make it difficult to wind down at the end of the day. Think about how a casino's lights keep you revved up," says Katherine Grace Morris, PhD, a psychologist in Maryland who specializes in making over people's home and work environments. Use spot lighting for areas where you need brightness, such as next to the sofa where you read, and put overhead lights on dimmers. Also, switch to full-spectrum bulbs, which mimic natural light better than standard ones do.

"They cost a bit more, but they're worth it because they create a more soothing natural atmosphere," says Dr. Morris.

Create pedestrian-friendly paths. "If you can barely get into a chair without banging your leg on the coffee table, or if the path from the sofa to the door is cramped, rearrange your furniture," says Roberts. "Not being able to safely and easily move about produces anxiety—not to mention an easy way to trip or stub a toe."

Simplify your color scheme. Use restraint with patterns and loud colors. If you mix patterns, keep their color schemes similar, and if you like lots of colors, keep patterns to a minimum.

"If you have too many bright colors or high-contrast patterns in a room, your eyes are going to be drawn all over the place, making it difficult to relax," says Dr. Morris. Simple designs and colors, on the other hand, are soothing. "The less-is-more rule applies to shelves and tabletops, too," adds Rien. "Don't fill them just because they're there. Instead, display just a few pieces that are meaningful."

Bring the outdoors in. Being surrounded by natural elements encourages friendlier interactions with others, found a University of Rochester study. For a more peaceful home, bring in a couple of houseplants or hang a mirror across from your largest window to maximize outdoor vantage points. If your view includes more buildings than trees, hang landscape photographs on the walls, says Roberts.

BEDROOMS

Use soothing hues. "Generally, we find cool shades of blue and green and neutral earth tones to be relaxing because they remind us of nature," says color expert Leatrice Eiseman, author of *Color: Messages and Meanings.* If you're not ready to commit to new paint, incorporate a few accessories, such as throw pillows, a quilt, or lamp shades, in calming colors.

Switch off electronics. To rest easier, remove all televisions and computers from your bedroom. The light emitted by these devices signals the brain to stay awake, interfering with a good night's sleep and leaving you with elevated levels of stress hormones in the morning. If you must keep these gadgets where you sleep, Rien recommends placing the TV in a cabinet and putting a screen between your bed and the computer.

Bring your fantasy to life. Think about what paradise looks like to you. If it's a tropical island, add sand and sea shades and tropical touches, such as wicker side tables or a sea grass rug. Prefer a mountain cabin or country home? Then add colors, textures, and accessories to your bedroom decor that call those settings to mind. "Design is highly individual, so mine your past experiences and flip through design magazines to identify what elements make a room feel relaxing to you," says Rien.

The Stress-Diabetes-Belly-Fat Triangle

When stress strikes, fight-or-flight hormones boost blood sugar and increase alertness. One, called cortisol, even triggers cravings for high-calorie foods and directs your body to store the excess calories as an "emergency fuel supply" in . . . you guessed it . . . belly fat.

In prehistoric days, this system helped cavemen outrun marauding predators and successfully bring home dinner after hunting. But it's no asset in the 21st century, when everything from a flat tire to a family emergency to a demanding boss leads to chronic stress and all of its negative health consequences. Lucky for us, scientists have also discovered an equal and opposite force that counteracts stress. In amazing real-world medical studies with real people (we're not talking test tubes or mice!), this "relaxation response" has reversed some of the worst effects of stress.

You've experienced this profoundly serene "Ah-h-h" if you've ever had a terrific massage, spent a week of perfect vacation time at the beach, or awakened after a night of long, peaceful slumber. Deep relaxation might steal upon you while cuddling in front of a fire with your kids, petting a beloved dog or cat, holding hands with a loved one, praying—or doing anything that brings bliss and contentment. The good news? You don't have to wait for it. You can invoke this level of deep, restoring calm whenever you need it.

Here's how vaporizing stress benefits your belly, your weight, your health.

Healthier blood sugar. In a breakthrough study conducted at Duke University, 108 women and men with type 2 diabetes took diabetes-education classes with or without stress management training. After a year, whereas A1c levels rose slightly in the control group, more than half of the stress relief group improved their blood sugar levels by at least 0.5 percent on an A1c test, a check of long-term blood sugar control. One-third reduced their A1c test result by 1 percentage point or more. That's huge: Lowering

come to believe that sharing our feelings is the only way to deal with life's struggles. But just the opposite is often true.

"We've long thought that talking about problems is always better, but there's also evidence suggesting that this coping style doesn't work for everybody," explains Karin Coifman, PhD, an assistant professor of clinical psychology at Kent State University. Dr. Coifman and colleagues looked at how people whose spouse or child had just died coped with their loss. They

your A1c levels that much cuts risk for diabetes-related complications such as heart disease, kidney failure, nerve damage, and vision problems by 17 to 35 percent. Study participants soothed their stress with muscle relaxation, deep breathing, and positive mental imagery.

Less insulin resistance. When researchers at the University of Virginia Health System in Charlottesville reviewed 70 studies on the health benefits of yoga—one of the ultimate relaxation exercises!—they discovered that this stress reducer can reverse insulin resistance. How much? Lead researcher Kim Innes, PhD, an assistant professor of research in the university's School of Nursing, found that yoga improved insulin sensitivity by about 19 percent. And it worked for a wide variety of people with and without diabetes, women and men, young and older.

Help for stress eating. A recent British study confirms something most of us already know up close and personal. It's easy—almost automatic—to reach for a snack when daily life becomes overwhelming or just plain annoying. Researchers at University College London found that stress snackers don't reach for baby carrots. They head for high-sugar, high-fat, high-calorie foods. (That explains why it's so easy to head for the vending machine and totally forget the apple in your purse when anxiety levels rise at work!) Practicing stress reduction lets you defuse rising tensions in the moment, leaving you feeling more relaxed and in control, and less likely to reach for the M&M's to feel better.

Easier weight loss. In a study of 225 overweight New Zealand women who followed one of three healthy lifestyle programs, only those who learned stress management strategies lost weight—5½ pounds. The women used a tension-melting progressive muscle relaxation technique, deep and slow abdominal breathing, and soothing visualizations.

learned that many of the subjects who avoided thinking or talking about their sadness—a style psychologists call repressive coping—had fewer short-term health problems, such as sore throats, diarrhea, and shortness of breath, as well as a lower incidence of long-term psychological problems. What's more, they returned to their everyday lives more quickly than those who dwelled upon their grief.

"There's a lot to be said for getting on with the business of living," says

Dr. Coifman. "People who talk endlessly about their problems are actually the ones at greater risk of depression." In fact, researchers at the University of Missouri, Columbia, found that participants who repeatedly expressed their sadness or disappointment were more likely to develop depression and anxiety. That doesn't mean you should just suck it up when something bad happens. While you shouldn't deny yourself natural grieving moments, learning to direct your attention away from the stressor is a powerful coping mechanism. So after experiencing that initial burst of tears, turn to something positive; check in on a friend or rearrange your furniture. It's an important skill to look beyond the bad. We wouldn't survive as a species otherwise, Dr. Coifman adds.

Yesterday's Wisdom: Never Soothe Yourself with Food

Today's smart strategy: Treat yourself to chocolate.

We've been warned that bingeing on cookies and ice cream is a poor way to ease a worried state of mind and can actually create more anxiety. But here's a sweet exception to the rule: Indulging in a little chocolate can actually help. According to new findings published in the *Journal of Proteome Research,* eating a few pieces of dark chocolate when you're feeling on edge can help calm your nerves. In the study, stressed-out participants who ate $1^1/_2$ ounces of dark chocolate a day for 2 weeks had reduced levels of stress hormones. We can't think of a better way to treat yourself to some dessert, guilt and stress free!

Yesterday's Wisdom: "Om" Your Way to Calmness

Today's smart strategy: Do something you love.

For some people, meditation is the secret to serenity, but for others, it's a fast track to frayed nerves. In fact, in a study published in the *Journal of Consulting and Clinical Psychology,* 54 percent of participants reported feeling anxious while meditating!

"There is no evidence that meditation 'cools off' the body's stress response better than any other type of stress reduction technique, so you have to find what works for you," insists Jonathan C. Smith, PhD, director of the Stress Institute at Roosevelt University. Anything that allows you to disengage from your thoughts can help you relax.

One way meditation works is by breaking the chain of everyday thoughts, which are often tied to our to-do lists and other stressors, according to Herbert Benson, MD, director emeritus of the Benson-Henry Institute for Mind Body Medicine at Massachusetts General Hospital in Boston and author of *Relaxation Revolution.* While chanting a mantra quiets your mind, if meditating is not your thing, any repetitive activity that keeps your attention in the present moment, including jogging, swimming, painting, or praying, will work just as well, he says.

19

Stay-Calm Solutions from Stress

SURVIVORS

New research on traumatized soldiers shows how damaging stress can be—and reveals five powerful tools that can help us all build resilience.

When most people think about post-traumatic stress disorder (PTSD), they think of soldiers, but PTSD can occur after anyone goes through a traumatic event like an assault or disaster. There has been a recent surge in PTSD research spurred not just by the wars in Iraq and Afghanistan but also by terrorism and natural disasters. Government institutions, military hospitals, and universities have all stepped up efforts to understand this anxiety disorder, teasing out what makes some people vulnerable and others resilient, as well as how the brain can heal. What they're discovering about PTSD is yielding important insights into how the rest of us can manage the moderate stress we deal with every day.

"The mind needs support—we call it 'mental armor'—just as much as the body does," says Amishi Jha, PhD, an associate professor of psychology at the University of Pennsylvania, who studies stress-fighting techniques such as mindfulness to help military personnel. "Research shows it's possible to cushion yourself against stress, and the tactics we're using with soldiers also apply to real folks and more common types of anxiety."

Key to the recent breakthroughs is a much clearer picture of how destructive stress can be. Persistent anxiety can kill neurons in brain structures concerned with memory and decision making, and such damage is even visible on brain scans.

Although women are less likely to experience traumatic events than men are (about half of women in the United States will encounter a trauma in their lifetime, most commonly sexual assault, followed by car crash), they are twice as likely to develop PTSD when they do, says the US Department of Veterans Affairs. Women are also more vulnerable to everyday stress. Mothers, for example, are five times as likely as fathers to rate their stress at the highest level, says the American Psychological Association.

Fortunately, experts are learning that all along the continuum—from severe anxiety disorders to garden-variety worry—coping and even prevention tactics are highly effective. Here's what new PTSD science can teach all of us about outsmarting stress. If these solutions work for soldiers in Iraq and Afghanistan, they can certainly help the rest of us on the home front.

For Stress Survivors: Build Mental Armor with Meditation

Mindfulness meditation works wonders to boost stress resilience, say experts from the University of Pennsylvania who are using the practice with military personnel.

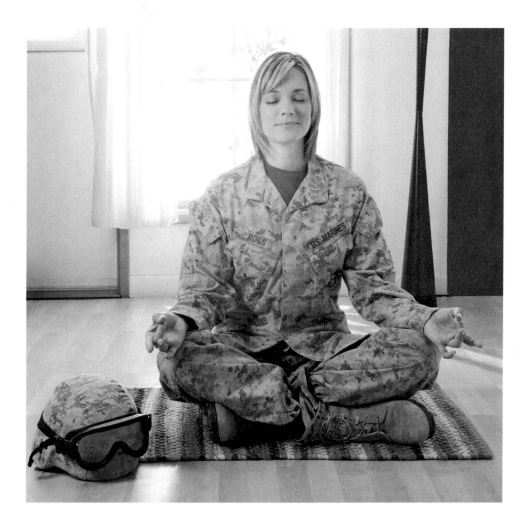

"We teach them to focus on the present moment instead of catastrophizing about the future," says Dr. Jha. After 8 weeks of meditation training, Marines became less reactive to stressors, and they were more alert and exhibited better memory.

FOR THE REST OF US: TAKE SHORT MINDFULNESS BREAKS

"Even I get too busy to meditate," says Dr. Jha. "Then I remember the Marines in the study calling my colleague while they were deployed to ask for mindfulness pointers, and I think, If they can do it in a war zone, I can do it in my office!"

Try this technique Marines use anywhere: Sit upright, focus on your breath, and pay attention to a physical sensation, such as the feel of air in your nostrils. When your mind wanders, notice the disruption, then return your attention to that simple sensation. Dr. Jha herself now meditates 5 to 10 minutes at a time, several times a day.

For Stress Survivors: Remember the Tough Stuff

Cognitive behavioral therapy (CBT)—which helps you recognize and change knee-jerk reactions to stress triggers—is one of the most effective methods of managing PTSD. In the military, such training can include a technique called "exposure therapy," in which soldiers relive disturbing past experiences in small doses with a therapist until the memories become less overwhelming. Along the same lines, doctors have achieved promising results by asking patients who developed PTSD following an illness to imagine a relapse.

Such intense visualizations should be undertaken only with a licensed professional, but "practicing" feeling stressed can help anyone cope day to day, says Elizabeth Carll, PhD, a trauma specialist on Long Island, New York. "If you learn to recognize how your body feels when anxiety starts, it's easier to intervene and calm yourself."

FOR THE REST OF US: IMAGINE A MOMENT OF TENSION

Fortify yourself against anxiety by trying an at-home exercise, says Susan Fletcher, PhD, a psychologist in private practice in Plano, Texas. Picture yourself in a stressful place, such as your commute, and imagine the tension you feel. Write out the realities of the situation: *If I don't leave by 7:30, I'll be late. On the other hand,* *I'll be in traffic about 60 minutes, so I can listen to a book on disc.* This lets you feel the stress and know it's not debilitating, and helps you devise solutions. If you want to try formal CBT, which encompasses a range of methods, you can find a certified practitioner through the National Association of Cognitive-Behavioral Therapists at www.nacbt.org.

For Stress Survivors: Bike for Long-Term Resilience

Researchers are learning that exercise doesn't just soothe stress, it also fortifies brain cells so they're less vulnerable to anxiety in the future. Neuroscientists at Princeton University recently discovered that neurons created in the brains of rats that run regularly are less stress-sensitive than those in rats that don't exercise.

While all exercise adds to your resilience, PTSD experts find that outdoor activities are particularly beneficial—especially cycling, says Melissa Puckett, a recreation therapist at the VA Palo Alto Healthcare System in California. "It's so effective because of the fresh air and the fact that it can be a group activity," she says. "We've seen people who were once afraid to leave the house make tremendous strides."

FOR THE REST OF US: SWEAT OUTSIDE FOR 5 MINUTES

Break from the gym and try something outdoorsy, like hiking or a simple walk.

Even 5 minutes outside—especially if spent near water, like a fountain or stream—is enough for a mental boost, found a 2010 study from the University of Essex in England.

For Stress Survivors: Pets Can Reduce Your Use of Meds

New research shows that owning an animal is an even more powerful way to cultivate calm than previously thought. An astonishing 82 percent of PTSD patients paired with a service dog reported a significant reduction in symptoms, and 40 percent were able to decrease their medications, in an ongoing study at the Walter Reed Army Medical Center. The specially trained pooches can sense when a panic attack is coming before their owners do, and then give them a nudge to start some preemptive deep breathing.

"While we don't yet understand why, we know the dogs' presence affects serotonin levels and the immune system," says lead study researcher Craig Love, PhD. "The animals are so helpful, one soldier named her dog Paxil."

FOR THE REST OF US: BOND WITH FIDO
Pet owners can reduce stress by building extra playtime into the day, says Dr. Carll. If you don't own a pet, offer to take a neighbor's dog for an after-dinner walk or cat-sit for a friend. Even short outings provide enough "pet exposure" to lessen anxiety.

ARE YOU STRESS PRONE?

The new PTSD research has made doctors increasingly adept at predicting who is at risk of developing the disorder, as well as everyday stress. The following factors indicate higher stress vulnerability.

- Negative life events such as divorce
- Low self-esteem
- Lack of a social support network
- Blaming yourself when things go wrong

Realizing you're more susceptible is a wake-up call; deploy antistress tactics if you find yourself doing the following.

- Acting overly emotional
- Feeling too tired to function
- Snapping at people
- Suffering headaches or stomach upset

For Stress Survivors: Sleep to Rebalance Sneaky Stress Hormones

Sleep suppresses stress hormones, such as cortisol, and spurs the release of others, like DHEA, which play a key role in resilience and protecting the body from stress. Yale University researchers tracked the hormone levels of a group of elite Special Forces soldiers who operate in treacherous underwater conditions and confirmed that higher DHEA levels predicted which divers were most stress hardy. Among women with PTSD, those with higher levels of DHEA have fewer negative moods, other Yale researchers found.

FOR THE REST OF US: DO A NIGHTLY STRESS SCAN

To boost DHEA naturally, get more sleep. Before you set your alarm, take stock of your stress status, says Dr. Fletcher. The more demanding your days, the more sleep you need to handle them. If the recommended 7 to 8 hours isn't possible, at least plan for an early night or two during a rough week or, if nothing else, a weekend nap.

"And get anything that reminds you of work—laundry, your laptop—out of your bedroom," Dr. Fletcher adds. "It's psychologically noisy."

These coping skills don't just make it easier to manage stress, they help you thrive in general. "People who beat chronic stress often develop positive shifts in their outlook," says Elissa Epel, PhD, a stress researcher at the University of California, San Francisco. Clichéd as it sounds, surviving a stressful event can open a new philosophical window on life. "People don't just cope, they grow," says Dr. Carll. "And the experience makes them stronger overall."

Snag more stress-soothing Zzzzs with the tips at www.prevention.com/100waystosleep.

20

Sleep: It Does a

BODY GOOD

Sleep has an effect on weight and blood sugar control. Here, three exhausted women fall asleep faster and sleep more soundly with the help of a top expert. Learn how you can get your Zzzs, too.

A good night's sleep is as easy as slipping under the covers and closing your eyes, right? If only. More than half of American women say they sleep well only a few nights a week, reports a National Sleep Foundation survey. Although this survey was on women, the results that they found and the lessons that they learned can also be applied to men.

"Sleep issues are common for women over 40—and usually very solvable," says sleep specialist Rubin Naiman, PhD, a clinical assistant professor of medicine at the University of Arizona's Center for Integrative Medicine. "With simple lifestyle changes, you can improve the quality of sleep, as well as mood and overall well-being." Here's how he helped three women get the shut-eye they need for optimal health and happiness.

Sleep Thief: Hyperactive Brain

Margot Tohn, 44, is a self-described over-achiever: On top of running her own publishing company, she takes care of her ailing father, volunteers for several charity organizations, and tries to play tennis with friends or go to the opera once a week. Her list of to-dos and obligations never ends, yet she often feels as though she's not doing enough. Even after she

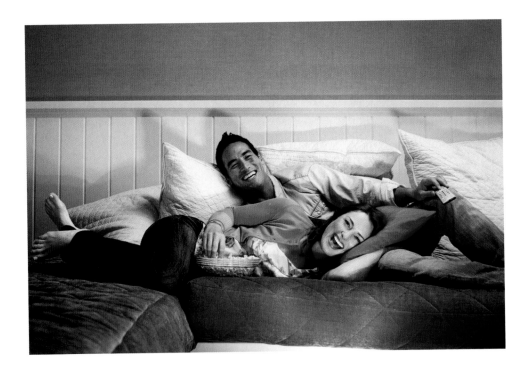

turns in for the night, her mind is still going, running through what she accomplished that day and planning for the next. She doesn't actually get to sleep until 1 to 2 a.m., then wakes at about 5:30, feeling anxious to get started. By the afternoon, Margot feels irritable and in desperate need of a nap.

OUR EXPERT SAYS

"This sleep problem is primarily psychological," explains Dr. Naiman. "Margot is entirely too hard on herself, and all that ruminating creates anxiety, which shifts the brain into high-alert mode instead of allowing it to wind down." When she starts to criticize herself or feel guilty about not running an errand right away for her family, for example, she needs to stop and think: Am I really hurting anyone by not doing this immediately? Taking a second to think rationally will help her calm down.

The other problem is that Margot's day is too jam-packed, adds Dr. Naiman. "She has no alone time to process her thoughts, so her mind essentially makes up for it at night." This pre-bed routine will help her mind and body relax.

Unplug an hour before bed. That includes the television, computer, cell phone, and any other glowing tech tools. Research shows that the brain misreads artificial light as daylight, so it doesn't release melatonin, a sleep-regulating chemical, which is normally triggered by darkness.

Take a warm shower or bath. Your body temperature goes down when you get out,

Do You Need a Sleep Pro?

If any of the following apply to you, talk with your doctor about getting evaluated for sleep apnea and other sleep disorders.

Are you constantly exhausted, even when you get 8 or more hours of sleep?

Do you have a hard time staying awake at work or while driving?

Has someone told you that you snore heavily or gasp for breath during your sleep?

which makes you feel sleepy. That's because it mimics what occurs deep inside the body at night, when internal temperature drops to its lowest level.

Meditate or pray for 10 minutes. Several studies show that it can help reduce anxiety, release negative thinking, and improve sleep. Sit quietly in a comfortable position and repeat a phrase you find relaxing, such as "Keep letting go."

HOW IT WORKED

"Though I'm not sleeping for 8 hours a night yet, the quality of my sleep has definitely improved because I'm much more energized during the day," Margot says. "The relaxation routine took me a little while to get used to: I never meditated before, so at first I could sit quietly for only

FIVE SURPRISING SIGNS YOU'RE SLEEP DEPRIVED

Our bodies give us plenty of signals when we're tired, but some of us are so used to being sleep deprived that we remain oblivious to how impaired we really are. Sleep debt isn't something you can pay off in a weekend, researchers say. It can take weeks of building up restorative sleep habits. In the meantime, here are some signs you might be sleep deprived. See "Your High-Energy Recovery Plan" on page 192 for temporary fixes while you get your sleep schedule back on track.

You're flummoxed by even simple decisions. You're up late one night booking your next vacation, and even though you know the dates and destination, you're overwhelmed by minor details. Should you get a refundable ticket? Window or aisle seat? Rent a car now or later? When you're tired, you're less able to distinguish between important and irrelevant information, such as your seat assignment, according to Sean Drummond, PhD, a sleep researcher at the University of California, San Diego. The result: Even the simplest decision takes on exaggerated importance.

Tired people also take riskier gambles to maximize results ("Maybe if I wait until the last minute, the ticket price will go down!") and have trouble adjusting to changing circumstances (such as firming up an itinerary if flying from an unfamiliar airport).

You've been eating all day and you're still hungry. Studies show that chronic sleep loss can disrupt blood sugar levels and cause the body to produce less leptin, a hormone that curbs appetite, and more ghrelin, leptin's hunger-stimulating counterpart. Because of these physiological changes, you might be more likely to overeat when you skimp on sleep, and the food you pick probably won't be either nutritious or a lasting source of energy. Tired people tend to be particularly drawn to sugars and other simple carbohydrates, probably because the body is looking for a quick pick-me-up, says Lisa Shives, MD, a spokesperson for the American Academy of Sleep Medicine. Sleep deprivation also tends to erode self-control, making you more likely to choose a brownie over carrot sticks.

You keep coming down with colds. People who get inadequate sleep are more vulnerable

---

about 2 minutes at a time. I eventually worked up to 10 minutes, and it does help ease my mind. I also take a hot shower at night and do a few stretches before I go to bed, which relaxes my body. Plus, I started to realize that my all-or-nothing attitude wasn't doing me any favors, so on nights when I get home late, I make sure to do my pre-bed routine for even just 10 to 20 minutes, instead of forgoing it entirely because I don't have a full hour."

KEY MOVE

Keep a journal. "I make a list each night of 10 things I am grateful for—from good friends to a good hair day," Margot says. "I

to infection than those who are well rested, says William Kohler, MD, medical director of the Florida Sleep Institute. In one study, researchers injected healthy volunteers with a cold virus. Those who slept less than 7 hours a night for the previous week were three times more likely to develop symptoms than those who got 8 hours or more. In another study, people who got only 4 hours of sleep for several nights in a row had a weaker immune response to the flu vaccine than those who slept between $7\frac{1}{2}$ and $8\frac{1}{2}$ hours.

The ballads on *American Idol* move you to tears. Don't automatically chalk up your sudden weepiness to PMS: Without sleep, you are more emotionally volatile. In one brain imaging study, for example, people who missed a night of sleep and viewed disturbing images had 60 percent more activity in the amygdala, which is involved in processing fear and anxiety, compared with better-rested volunteers. The study also found that the sleepy volunteers' amygdala communicated less with the part of the brain that determines appropriate emotional responses, suggesting that they weren't doing a good job of tempering their emotions.

When we're sleep deprived, we might also feel glum because tired brains store negative memories more effectively than positive or neutral ones. As a result of all this, Dr. Shives says, "If you are chronically sleep deprived, you could act like someone with depression."

You've become a klutz. One moment you're brewing a cup of afternoon tea and the next thing you know you've spilled it all over yourself. Researchers have accumulated ample evidence that the sleep deprived have slower and less precise motor skills, but exactly why isn't yet known, says Clete Kushida, MD, PhD, director of Stanford University Center for Human Sleep Research. Sleepy people may be clumsier for several reasons: Impaired reflexes and a lack of focus might make it hard for them to react quickly enough to things that spring up in their path.

Another possibility: Sleepiness throws off balance or depth perception. In any case, it's not uncommon for very sleepy people to black out momentarily when the body's urge to sleep gets too strong. So it's possible that your klutziness stems from "microsleeps" that last for a second or two, Dr. Kushida says—just long enough to trip on the curb or drop a glass.

feel less anxious when I take a few minutes to focus on how much I'm blessed."

Sleep Thief: Waking Up Four Times a Night

Virginia Camasca, 40, has battled insomnia for 5 years, trying all sorts of things from herbs to special diets with no success. At night, she spends up to an hour trying to get comfortable before eventually dozing off, but then she wakes up several times before the alarm rings—often to use the bathroom, sometimes just because. She used to dream frequently but now rarely does, which some research

Your High-Energy Recovery Plan

To erase your sleep debt (it may take several weeks), aim for 7 to 8 hours of sleep every night. Meanwhile, here's how to suppress daytime fogginess, stay alert, and get deeper Zzzs.

In the morning, soak up the sun. Morning rays boost energy by suppressing the sleepiness-inducing hormone melatonin. An early morning walk will help synchronize your internal clock to the sun, averting an energy slump in the afternoon.

After lunch, time your nap. Research shows that naps, especially power naps of 20 to 30 minutes, help ward off fatigue. To maximize the benefits, try to take a siesta after lunch, when your energy levels are particularly low. Limit rest to less than 30 minutes, or stretch it out to 60 to 90 minutes to avoid grogginess that results from waking up in the middle of deep sleep.

In the early evening, reenergize with exercise. Even though you're tired, forcing yourself to do aerobic exercise will energize you for a couple of hours and make it easier to fall asleep at night. Your body temperature naturally falls at night, shortly before bedtime, so the natural dip in temperature that happens about 2 hours after a workout can help you get to bed at a decent hour and wake up refreshed the next morning.

awake if I get up in the middle of the night. That way, I'm less stressed if I wake up, so it's easier to drift off again."

Sleep Thief: Night Sweats and Heavy Snoring

Tracy Lobdell, 52, has gained more than 50 pounds over the past 5 years, and it's taking a toll on her sleep habits. She snores heavily and suspects she may have sleep apnea, a serious condition that occurs when a person stops breathing for seconds at a time because of airway obstructions, which are often caused or made worse by excess body fat. She recently lost a few pounds by adopting a healthier diet and practicing portion control, but she never has the time or energy to exercise. Tracy is also in the throes of menopause and suffers from hot flashes and night sweats. Plus, her husband and dog—both of whom share her bed—snore, too, and there's barely room for the three of them on their queen-size mattress. The result: Tracy tosses and turns all

All day, work on something interesting. Even tired people pay better attention to tasks they find mentally stimulating. So even though you might be tempted to go for the mindless stuff—filing, folding laundry—you'll be more alert if you pick a project that intrigues you.

Each meal and snack, eat for stamina. Big meals and high-sugar foods can cause blood sugar to spike then plummet, so every few hours while you're recovering eat a snack (about 100 calories), or try smaller meals (of no more than 400 calories) that contain complex carbohydrates, some protein, and a small amount of healthy fat. Try a handful of nuts or reduced-fat cheese and crackers at low-energy times of the day—typically, early morning and late afternoon.

As needed, boost your caffeine. Sugary "energy drinks" can be hidden calorie traps, but researchers think there is something about the combination of sugar and caffeine that makes people more alert than caffeine alone. Next time you are feeling particularly brain-dead, add a tablespoon of honey to your tea or stir a spoonful of sugar into your espresso. To keep yourself from reaching that state to begin with, try divvying up your one big mug of coffee in the morning into several coffee breaks throughout the day.

night and is moody, unproductive, and tired during the day.

OUR EXPERT SAYS

"Severe snoring, weight gain, and significant daytime drowsiness all indicate possible sleep apnea," says Dr. Naiman. "But even if Tracy doesn't have the condition, snoring can make it difficult for her to get into the deep stages of sleep." Although it's a good idea for her to get tested for apnea, Tracy can help ease snoring and other possible apnea symp-

toms by keeping up the weight loss. To slim down even faster, she should add 30 minutes of aerobic exercise to her routine 5 or 6 days a week, says Dr. Naiman. Shedding extra pounds might ease night sweats, too. And to sleep more soundly, she should try these bedtime tweaks.

Switch to the side. Sleeping on the back, as Tracy does now, isn't ideal for heavy snorers or people with apnea. It allows the soft palate to hang in a direction that can obstruct breathing. Sleeping on either side, however, opens up airways to

Sleep! It's Nonnegotiable

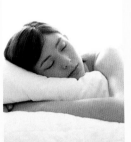

A good night's sleep isn't just about hitting the ground running in the morning. If you get the 7 to 9 hours experts advise, you can expect the following added benefits.

Lower risk of heart disease and diabetes. Lack of sleep is associated with higher levels of stress hormones that may raise blood pressure and affect glucose metabolism. A new study found that the risk for high blood pressure among insomniacs who slept less than 5 hours per night was five times greater than among those who logged more than 6 hours. They were also three times likelier to have diabetes, compared with those without insomnia who slept more than 6 hours.

Fewer sniffles. People who get less than 7 hours per night are three times likelier to catch colds, according to a *JAMA* study. Reason: Sleep boosts immunity, and too little sleep impairs it.

A trimmer waistline. People who logged 7 to 9 hours a night had an average BMI of 24.8, almost 2 points lower than the average BMI of those who slept less, University of Washington researchers found. Too little sleep may throw off hormones that regulate appetite.

alleviate breathing issues. To help stay in this position, Dr. Naiman suggests propping one pillow behind your back and another in front of your waist.

Make the bed a pet-free zone. Tuck the pooch into a doggie bed in another room. When Tracy shares her sleeping space with her pet, it gives her little room to move, and though she might not realize it, her dog's fidgeting and kicking wake her throughout the night.

Keep the bedroom cool. Exactly how cool depends on your preference, but Dr. Naiman suggests around 68°F. Wear lightweight pajamas and cover up with a sheet instead of a blanket. This will help reduce the severity of night sweats.

HOW IT WORKED

"For the first time in years, I actually feel well rested," Tracy says. "I plan to get tested for apnea, but I'm already falling asleep much faster and my hot flashes are less frequent and severe. I even got used to sleeping on my side. The toughest part for me was making my dog sleep in the other room. I felt guilty, but it really is so much more comfortable. Instead, I let her spend 10 minutes in bed with me in the morning. I think of it as trading quantity for quality. I've continued to lose weight by watching my diet. I've dropped 10 pounds and counting. I haven't made time for exercise yet, but I definitely have more energy now, so it's next on my list."

KEY MOVE

Cut back caffeine. "I used to drink about six glasses of iced black and orange tea every day," Tracy says. "Dr. Naiman suggested that I switch to decaf or 100 percent iced green tea, which can have half as much caffeine. Now in the mornings I

FOUR WAYS TO SLEEP MORE DEEPLY

Here's how to hit the hay earlier.

- Gradually advance your bedtime by 15 minutes a night.
- Dim the lights in your home about an hour before bed, and start a routine that tells your body it's time to snooze (put on pajamas, brush teeth, wash face).
- Avoid the TV and computer.
- Meditate or do light stretching. People who relax in the evening fall asleep about 30 minutes sooner than those who don't and get an extra hour of sleep.

have a little black and orange tea, but in the afternoon, I stick to green. I actually don't miss the caffeine at all."

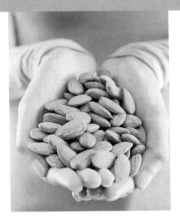
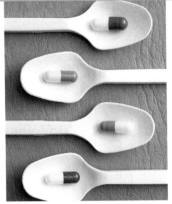
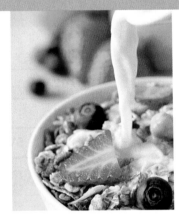

COMPLICATIONS
Medical Breakthroughs

Diabetes increases your risk for many serious health problems, such as heart disease, high blood pressure, eye complications, even Alzheimer's disease and depression. Here's the good news: With the correct treatment and recommended lifestyle changes, many people with diabetes are able to prevent or delay the onset of complications.

▨ DISEASE-PROOF YOUR DIET

Similar foods can contain drastically different nutrient levels. Are your picks protecting your health as well as they could? Test yourself.

Which is the best food . . .

1. . . .to lower cholesterol? Red bell pepper or green bell pepper?

2. . . .to prevent dementia? Almonds or peanuts?

3. . . .to ward off hearing loss? Broccoli or spinach?

4. . . .to maintain a healthy blood pressure? Low-fat yogurt or cottage cheese?

ANSWERS

1. Red bell pepper for a double dose of heart-healthy vitamin C. A recent study found that 500 milligrams daily can significantly reduce bad LDL cholesterol and triglycerides.

2. Almonds for three times the vitamin E. Getting about 8 milligrams daily can help lower your risk of Alzheimer's disease by 67 percent.

3. Spinach for twice as much folate. A study of 26,273 men found that a high intake can reduce your risk of hearing loss by 20 percent.

4. Low-fat yogurt for three times the calcium. Getting 1,000 to 1,200 milligrams daily can help reduce blood pressure by up to 40 percent, according to researchers.

▨ CONSIDER THESE SUPPLEMENTS

Registered dietitians are better than most at meeting their nutritional needs with whole foods, but even they have dietary gaps. That's why 96 percent take at least one supplement, according to a new survey. Here's how they cover their bases.

- 84 percent take a multivitamin to support overall health.

- 63 percent take calcium to build and maintain strong bones.

- 47 percent take fish oil to ward off dementia and heart disease.

- 43 percent take vitamin D to fight cancer.

- 29 percent take vitamin C to boost immunity.

▨ TRY THIS AT HOME

Don't be surprised if your doctor's next order is to check your blood pressure yourself, because it pays to strap on the cuff. In a recent Finnish study, home blood pressure readings better predicted heart attacks and strokes than did readings at the doctor's office. The latter tend to be artificially elevated—known as white-coat hypertension—because the setting makes people tense up (on average, home tests were 8/3 mm Hg lower). Take your blood pressure twice a day—morning and night—for a week and average the results. Do this every 3 months, before a doctor visit, and after any changes in medications or lifestyle, or if you lose 15 pounds.

Try it. All the cardiologists we spoke to recommended Omron arm cuffs. Wrist or finger monitors are notoriously inaccurate. Try Omron BP760, $90, available at www.omronwebstore.com. This cuff can expand to fit any size arm, which is key to an accurate measure.

Expert tip. Always bring a new blood pressure monitor to your doctor to make sure it works before you start at-home readings.

▣ TEST YOURSELF

Here are two simple tests for heart disease you can take yourself, at home.

How flexible are you? Adults over age 40 who were the most limber had 30 percent less stiffness in the arteries than less-flexible participants in a recent Japanese study. Stretching for 10 to 15 minutes a day may keep arteries pliable. They might be affected by the elasticity of the muscles and tissue that surround them.

The average reduction in systolic blood pressure on a low-salt diet.

23

What's your waist-to-height ratio? The size of your abdominal fat cells may be the best indicator of your type 2 diabetes risk, found new Swedish research. Diabetes increases your odds of stroke and death from heart disease by two to four times. The size of your waistline relative to your height is the most accurate way to gauge abdominal fat. Measure your waist, then divide by your height (in inches). Aim for a waist-to-height ratio of less than 0.5.

▣ LOWER YOUR CHOLESTEROL

Even moderately high cholesterol levels at midlife can significantly increase the risk of Alzheimer's disease and other forms of dementia decades later, according to a new study. Researchers found that people with borderline total cholesterol levels in middle age (200 to 239 milligrams per deciliter) were 50 percent more likely to develop vascular dementia compared with people with total cholesterol levels less than 200 mg/dl. But remember that several factors contribute to dementia, says study author and Finnish neurologist Alina Solomon, MD. "Cholesterol is a big part of the puzzle, but just one piece." It's also important to exercise, avoid high blood sugar, and engage in mentally challenging leisure activities.

▣ MEDITATE FOR YOUR HEART

Heart disease patients who practiced transcendental meditation twice a day were 47 percent less likely to experience heart attack, stroke, and death over a 5-year period, compared with a control group that took classes on healthy eating and exercise. Transcendental meditation's benefit is so powerful, it's comparable to a new class of heart disease–preventing drugs, says study author Robert Schneider, MD, director of the Institute for Natural Medicine and Prevention in Fairfield, Iowa.

21

Ancient Body,

MODERN LIFE

Here's why the blood sugar mismatch can lead to diabetes complications.

L ike a jewel-encrusted Fabergé egg or a vintage 1953 Studebaker, your body's system for managing blood sugar is a beautiful anachronism. Built to withstand the frequent famines, scarce feasts, and heavy physical demands of Stone Age life, it's out of place in a 21st-century landscape of Cinnabons, stuffed-crust pizza, and pay-per-view. Your body lives by prehistoric rules designed to keep mind and body running oh-so-frugally on a sometimes meager supply of glucose. It extracts every molecule of sugar from the foods you eat, then conserves precious glucose by hoarding the energy in muscle and liver cells for the times you need it most.

Yet Twinkies have replaced wild raspberries, and grain-fed beef and supersize fries have replaced freshly dug roots and lean wild game rich in good fat. Calorie consumption has soared, and daily exercise means walking from the front door to the car, not a 15-mile trek to the next watering hole.

The world has changed; our bodies have not. A growing stack of research links that fundamental mismatch to an amazing variety of modern-day blood sugar–related health problems, including heart attack, stroke, high blood pressure, diabetes, cancer, infertility, and even Alzheimer's disease, as well as birth defects, sexual dysfunction, blindness, kidney failure, and amputation. Even more alarming: The workings of this ancient sugar control system can put you at high risk for serious conditions even if your blood sugar levels look normal. Of course, risk rises higher if sugar levels soar into the prediabetic range, and higher still if you develop full-blown type 2 diabetes.

From Insulin Resistance to Diabetes

The problem isn't just sugar. Insulin, the hormone that tells cells to absorb blood sugar, plays a major role, too. In tiny amounts, this powerful protein is healthy and essential. But if inactivity, belly fat, and a high-fat, high-sugar diet have made your cells insulin resistant, a condition affecting as many as one in two American adults, your body pumps out two to three times more insulin than normal in order to force sugar into cells. The ploy works. Your cells receive the sugar they need (and your blood sugar levels will look normal on a fasting blood sugar test). But the excess insulin can raise your blood pressure, clog your arteries, over-tax your pancreas (raising diabetes risk), promote the growth of cancer cells, stop ovulation, and dim memory.

Once this hidden high blood sugar begins to do its damage, you develop a condition called metabolic syndrome, in

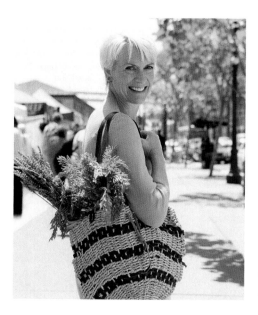

which biochemical changes triggered by insulin resistance begin to alter systems throughout your body. Metabolic syndrome can simmer undetected for decades. Blood sugar levels will rise into prediabetic and then diabetic zones if your pancreas can no longer produce enough insulin to overcome insulin resistance.

Diabetes adds new health risks, including vision problems, kidney failure, and bodywide nerve damage. A sobering new finding: These complications may begin to develop when your blood sugar is still in the prediabetic range (100 to 125 milligrams of glucose per deciliter of blood on a fasting blood sugar test).

"The complications of diabetes may begin years before diagnosis and much earlier than we thought," said Richard Kahn, PhD, chief scientific and medical officer for the American Diabetes Association. "That is really the big news, because we have not known when the changes start to occur."

Here's more of the latest research on the profound links between blood sugar control and your health.

Heart Disease and Stroke

In a Swedish study that tracked 1,826 people for 20 years, researchers found that those with metabolic syndrome had a 69 percent higher risk for heart attack than those without it. Others estimate that metabolic syndrome could sometimes triple heart risk. Diabetes magnifies the problem, as high glucose levels further assault arteries. People with diabetes are four times more likely to have a heart attack or stroke and are more likely to die than people who don't have diabetes, say Harvard Medical School researchers. Atherosclerosis accounts for virtually 80 percent of all deaths among diabetes patients.

High insulin levels turn your blood into a superhighway for bad fats—raising triglycerides; lowering good HDL cholesterol, the kind that mops up artery-choking LDL cholesterol; and making nasty LDL extra small and better able to invade artery walls. They raise levels of fibrinogen, which makes blood clot, and up your risk for high blood pressure by altering the way your kidneys process sodium. People with metabolic syndrome also have signs of more chronic, low-level inflammation, as if their

HIGH STAKES

A growing stack of research confirms that keeping your A1c level in a healthy range (experts recommend a reading of 6.5 to 7 percent for people with diabetes, lower if possible) is a powerful, effective strategy for sidestepping a host of serious, scary complications. This test measures average blood sugar for the last 2 to 3 months. Here's how a high A1c threatens your health.

Heart trouble. In a recent British study of 10,232 women and men with type 2 diabetes, University of Cambridge researchers found that every 1-point increase in A1c levels raised heart disease risk 24 percent for men and 28 percent for women. Other research shows that it doubles heart failure risk.

Brain attacks. The same study found that stroke risk rose 30 percent when A1c levels rose above 7 and tripled at levels above 10.

Amputation. Tulane University scientists found in a recent study of 4,526 women and men that an A1c over 7 triples the risk for peripheral vascular disease, the nerve damage responsible for foot and leg amputations among people with diabetes.

Blindness. In a study of 11,247 women and men, researchers from the International Diabetes Institute found that the odds for retinopathy—damage to the tiny blood vessels inside the retina—rose 25 percent when A1c levels were over 7.5 percent for up to 4 years, and 50 percent when A1c remained high more than 8 years.

Kidney damage and failure. The higher your A1c, the greater the odds for kidney failure, say Israeli researchers, who found that high blood sugar, high blood pressure, and high cholesterol levels all raise kidney risk for people with diabetes.

The bright side. You're in control. University of Oxford scientists say that reducing your A1c by tightening your blood sugar control cuts all these risks dramatically. A 1-point drop in your A1c level will reduce heart attack risk 14 percent, lower heart failure risk 16 percent, cut stroke risk 21 percent, cut risk for amputation resulting from peripheral vascular disease by 41 percent, and reduce risk for blindness or kidney failure by 35 percent.

immune systems are constantly on alert. This churns out compounds such as C-reactive protein that help pack extra fatty gunk into artery walls and raise the risk for heart-stopping blood clots.

Type 2 Diabetes

One in three people with metabolic syndrome will go on to develop type 2 diabetes.

The turning point may be encoded in your DNA.

Researchers from Iceland's Decode deCODE Genetics, a gene research company, recently announced the discovery of a "diabetes gene" carried by an astonishing 45 percent of humans around the world. The gene alone can't doom you to a diabetic future; experts say lifestyle pulls the trigger. A genetic "weakness" can prompt overtaxed insulin-producing cells in your pancreas to burn out, allowing blood sugar to rise.

Cancer

The link between insulin and cancer keeps getting stronger. High insulin levels tripled risk for breast cancer in a surprising University of Toronto study of 198 women. And among women with breast cancer, those with the highest levels were three times more likely to see cancer recur.

Researchers are also finding links between high insulin and prostate and colon cancer. National Cancer Institute scientists recently documented a doubled risk for pancreatic cancer among smokers with type 2 diabetes who had the highest levels of insulin and the most insulin resistance.

Insulin acts as a growth factor, making cancer cells grow quickly and divide wildly, says breast cancer researcher Pamela Goodwin, MD, of Toronto's Mount Sinai Hospital. Some cancer cells have more insulin receptors than normal cells do, allowing the hormone to dock easily.

Infertility and Birth Defects

Women with an infertility problem called polycystic ovary syndrome (PCOS) have insulin resistance and higher than normal insulin levels. While high insulin isn't the only cause, it's a major factor and helps explain why half of all women with PCOS develop diabetes by age 40 and 40 percent have signs of seriously clogged arteries by age 45.

In PCOS, high insulin may disrupt ovulation and prompt miscarriages by signaling a woman's ovaries to produce extra male hormones, says infertility specialist Sandra Carson, MD, a reproductive endocrinologist at Baylor College of Medicine in Houston. Signs of PCOS include menstrual periods that are more than 6 weeks apart, stubborn weight gain, acne, and abnormal facial or body hair.

Meanwhile, having diabetes before pregnancy can raise your baby's risk of birth defects—especially of the heart and spinal cord—two to five times higher than normal. Developing diabetes during pregnancy, a condition called gestational diabetes, raises your odds of delivering a high-birth-weight baby and developing preeclampsia, a dangerous pregnancy-related elevation in blood pressure.

Dementia and Alzheimer's Disease

Both overweight and diabetes increase the odds for dementia. Now researchers think insulin resistance in brain cells is one reason why.

In lab studies at the Joslin Diabetes Center in Boston, researchers found that the brain cells of insulin-resistant mice produced a protein also found in the brain lesions of people with Alzheimer's disease. Diabetes and insulin resistance may also shortchange a brain region responsible for memory—in some cases shrinking it significantly, research shows.

Vision Problems and Blindness

If you have diabetes or even prediabetes, high blood sugar levels can damage and destroy tiny capillaries in the eyes. The capillaries swell and weaken, clog, and burst—a condition called diabetic retinopathy that blurs vision and often leads to blindness. Diabetes is the leading cause of blindness in adults age 20 and up.

Also, chronically high blood sugar levels activate a substance called protein kinase C, which causes abnormal production of new blood vessels in the eye. The problem is, you don't need these new vessels, and they're more prone to leaking and bursting.

Nerve Damage and Amputation

About 70 percent of lower-leg amputations performed in 2003 were on people with diabetes, says the US Agency for Healthcare Research and Quality. The cause: high blood glucose that damages nerves and reduces circulation, making even the smallest cut or blister potentially a wound that won't heal.

Nerve damage can also cause impotence, arousal and orgasm difficulty for women, out-of-rhythm heartbeats, slowed digestion, and urinary problems.

Teeth

High blood sugar presents a triple threat to good oral health. First, it compromises your ability to fight infection, so even a small cold sore or tiny pocket of bacteria below the gum line could lead to serious trouble. Second, it raises the level of glucose in saliva. This "sweeter" saliva supports the growth of fungal (thrush) and bacterial infections. Third, high blood sugar can dry up saliva, leaving you with less of this vital infection-fighting moisture when you need it most.

The damage? In a new Italian study of 212 patients at the Dental Institute of the University of Sassari, researchers found three times more gum-disease bacteria in the mouths of people with diabetes than in those without diabetes. People with diabetes also had more dental plaque, more bleeding gums, and deeper openings at the gum line around each tooth, which is a sign of gum disease.

22

14 Ways Never to

GET CANCER

People with diabetes are more likely to develop cancer.
Good news: The following healthful lifestyle choices can
dramatically lower your risk.

F

irst, the good news: that is, if you have a healthy lifestyle.

"As many as 70 percent of known causes of cancers are avoidable and related to lifestyle," says Thomas A. Sellers, PhD, associate director for cancer prevention and control at Moffitt Cancer Center in Tampa. Diet, exercise, and avoidance of tobacco products are, of course, your first line of defense, but recent research has uncovered many small, surprising ways you can weave even more disease prevention into your everyday life. Try these novel strategies and your risk could dwindle even more.

Filter your tap water.

You'll reduce your exposure to known or suspected carcinogens and hormone-disrupting chemicals. A recent report from the President's Cancer Panel on how to reduce exposure to carcinogens suggests that home-filtered tap water is a safer bet than bottled water, whose quality often is not higher—and in some cases is worse—than water from municipal sources, according to a study by the Environmental Working Group. (*Consumer Reports'* top picks for faucet-mounted filters: Culligan, Pur Vertical, and the Brita OPFF-100.) Store water in stainless steel or glass to avoid chemical contaminants such as

the BPA that can leach from plastic bottles.

Stop topping your tank.

So say the EPA and the President's Cancer Panel: Pumping one last squirt of gas into your car after the nozzle clicks off can spill fuel and foil the pump's vapor recovery system, designed to keep toxic chemicals such as cancer-causing benzene out of the air, where they can come in contact with your skin or get into your lungs.

Marinate meat before grilling.

Processed, charred, and well-done meats can contain cancer-causing heterocyclic amines, which form when meat is seared at high temperatures, and polycyclic aromatic hydrocarbons, which get into food when it's charcoal broiled.

"The recommendation to cut down on grilled meat has really solid scientific evidence behind it," says Cheryl Lyn Walker, PhD, a professor of carcinogenesis at the University of Texas M. D. Anderson Cancer Center. If you do grill, add rosemary and thyme to your favorite marinade and soak meat for at least an hour before cooking. The antioxidant-rich spices can cut HCAs by as much as 87 percent, according to research at Kansas State University.

Caffeinate every day.

Java lovers who drank five or more cups of caffeinated coffee a day had a 40 percent decreased risk of brain cancer compared with people who drank the least, says a 2010 British study. A five-cup-a-day coffee habit reduces risks of cancers of the pharynx and mouth almost as much. Researchers credit the caffeine: Decaf had no comparable effect. But coffee was a more potent protector against these cancers than tea, which the British researchers said also offered protection against brain cancer.

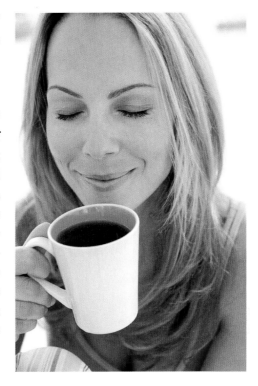

Water down your risks.

Drinking plenty of water and other liquids might reduce the risk of bladder cancer by diluting the concentration of cancer-causing agents in urine and helping to flush them through the bladder faster.

SPECIAL ALERT FOR WOMEN WITH BONE LOSS

If you have osteoporosis, your drug treatment may raise your risk of cancer of the esophagus (the tube that connects your mouth to your stomach). People who used bisphosphonate drugs like Fosamax for about 5 years had double the esophageal cancer risk, a recent study found, an increase likely related to side effects like stomach upset and esophageal inflammation.

"Your overall odds of esophageal cancer are still extremely low," says Barbara Burtness, MD, a professor of medical oncology at Fox Chase Cancer Center in Philadelphia. About 16,640 cases are diagnosed a year, and it's three to four times more common in men than in women. But if you have risk factors for esophageal cancer—smoking, drinking, acid reflux, or being overweight—ask your doctor about other bone-boosting options. He may prescribe the drug as a once-a-year intravenous dose, which should eliminate the esophageal cancer risk.

Switch to Powerhouse Foods

You get the biggest health benefit out of fruits and vegetables when you eat lots of different kinds. Yet most of us derive cancer-fighting phytonutrients from a handful of tried-and-true standbys that aren't always the most potent sources, according to a study presented at the 2010 Experimental Biology meeting, an annual gathering hosted by several research organizations. Here are some typical choices and better substitutes.

Cancer Fighter	Usual Source	Better Choice
Beta-carotene	Carrots	Sweet potatoes have double the beta-carotene of carrots.
Beta-cryptoxanthin	Oranges	One serving of papaya has 11 times more beta-cryptoxanthin than an orange and six times more than a cup of orange juice.
Lutein/zeaxanthin	Spinach	Cooked kale has seven times the lutein/zeaxanthin of raw spinach.
Ellagic acid	Strawberries	Fresh raspberries have three times more ellagic acid than strawberries do.
Glucosinolates	Broccoli	A half cup of Brussels sprouts contains four times more of these cancer-curbing compounds than the same amount of broccoli.

Drink at least 8 cups of liquid a day, suggests the American Cancer Society.

Load up on really green greens.

Next time you're choosing salad fixings, reach for the darkest varieties. The chlorophyll that gives them their color is loaded with magnesium, which some large studies have found lowers the risk of colon cancer in women.

"Magnesium affects signaling in cells, and without the right amount, cells may do things like divide and replicate when they shouldn't," says Dr. Walker. Just $1/2$ cup of cooked spinach provides 75 milligrams of magnesium, 20 percent of the daily value.

Snack on Brazil nuts.

They're a stellar source of selenium, an antioxidant that lowers the risk of bladder cancer in women, according to research from Dartmouth Medical School. Other studies have found that people with high blood levels of selenium have lower rates of dying from lung and colorectal cancers. Researchers think selenium protects cells from free radical damage, and it might also enhance immune function and suppress formation of blood vessels that nourish tumors.

Burn off this breast cancer risk factor.

Moderate exercise such as brisk walking 2 hours a week cuts risk of breast cancer 18 percent. Regular workouts may lower your risks by helping you burn fat, which otherwise produces its own estrogen, a known contributor to cancer.

Ask your doctor about breast density.

Women whose mammograms have revealed breast density readings of 75 percent or more have a cancer risk four to five times higher than that of women with low density scores, according to recent research. One theory is that denser breasts result from higher levels of estrogen, making exercise particularly important.

"Shrinking your body fat also changes growth factors, signaling proteins such as adipokines and hormones like insulin in ways that tend to turn off cancer-promoting processes in cells," Dr. Walker says.

Skip the dry cleaner.

A solvent known as perc (short for perchloroethylene) that's used in traditional dry cleaning may cause liver and kidney cancers and leukemia, according to a US Environmental Protection Agency finding backed in early 2010 by the National Academies of Science. The main dangers are to workers who handle chemicals or treated clothes using older machines, although experts have not concluded that consumers are also at increased cancer risk. Less toxic alternatives: Hand wash clothes with mild soap and air-dry them, spot cleaning if necessary with white vinegar.

Head off cell phone risks.

Use your cell phone only for short calls or texts, or use a hands-free device that keeps the phone—and the radio frequency energy it emits—away from your head. The point is more to preempt any risk than to protect against a proven danger. Evidence that cell phones increase brain cancer risk is "neither consistent nor conclusive," says the President's Cancer Panel report. But a number of review studies suggest there's a link.

Block the sun with color.

Choosing your outdoor outfit wisely may help protect against skin cancer, say Spanish scientists. In their research, blue and red fabrics offered significantly better protection against the sun's UV rays than white and yellow ones did.

Don't forget to put on a hat: Though melanoma can appear anywhere on the body, it's more common in areas the sun hits, and University of North Carolina at Chapel Hill researchers have found that people with melanomas on the scalp or neck die at almost twice the rate of people with the cancer on other areas of the body.

Eat clean foods.

The President's Cancer Panel recommends buying meat free of antibiotics and added hormones, which are suspected of causing endocrine problems, including cancer. The report also advises that you purchase produce grown without pesticides or wash conventionally grown food thoroughly to remove residues. (The foods with the most pesticides are celery, peaches, strawberries, apples, and blueberries.) "At least 40 known carcinogens are found in pesticides, and we should absolutely try to reduce exposure," Dr. Sellers says.

23

THE HEART

Attack You're about to Have

. . . will happen when you least expect it, over the course of an ordinary day, perhaps soon after you've gotten a clean bill of health from your doctor.

Y ou will be shocked. But you shouldn't be.

Here's a cutting-edge, your-life-depends-on-it plan to help you prevent the #1 killer of women and men.

Surprising Faces of Heart Attack

The following three women didn't think they were at high risk. Their stories are proof that you could be in danger without even knowing it.

NIKI LEFEVRE

Niki, 44, is a physical education teacher in Allentown, Pennsylvania.

A 5-foot-5, 115-pound triathlete, Niki considered herself so healthy that she used to joke about it. "I'd tell my husband, 'You're going to be stuck with me until I'm 115 years old.'" When she woke up with severe back pain last April, she figured it was a muscle spasm from training too hard for an upcoming race and headed off to work.

While she was playing tennis in her last-period gym class, the pain spread to her chest. "It hurt terribly to swing," she says. "I told the students, 'You've got to play me next week when I'm not feeling so bad. If I didn't know better, I'd say I was having a heart attack.'"

But she still got in her car to drive home. While talking to her husband on the way, she suddenly felt much worse and told him to call 911. "I was nauseated, sweating, and so light-headed that I pulled off the highway," she says. When the EMTs arrived 5 minutes later, they checked her pulse and blood pressure—both of which were low—and gave her oxygen. She blacked out.

At the hospital, the cardiologist took one look at her EKG and rushed her to the catheterization lab, where he inserted a stent. "He said if I hadn't been in such good shape, I would have died on the tennis court, because one of my main arteries was 100 percent blocked," she says. "I was sobbing, because I thought my life would never be the same again." Her annual checkups had never revealed high cholesterol or blood pressure, and she had no family history of heart disease.

But there was another problem: Nine years earlier, Niki had been diagnosed with hypersomnia, a rare sleep disorder. She needs 10 to 12 hours of sleep each night to feel "normal," but most nights she'd been getting less than 5, which more than doubles the risk of a heart attack, even in otherwise healthy people. Chronic sleep deprivation is more hazardous to women than to men, raising blood pressure and reducing the body's sensitivity to insulin, both of which can damage blood

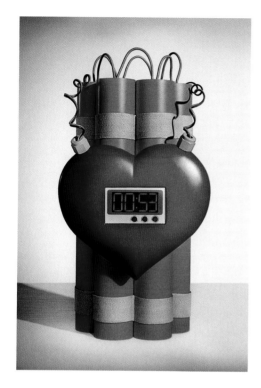

"I was worried about how we'd pay the mortgage," she says. Besides, she'd had trouble breathing before. "I passed out and fell down a flight of stairs at my doctor's office," she says. "He said it was an anxiety attack."

Her coworkers weren't concerned either—not even when the 245-pound King got so dizzy that she lay down on the floor by her desk. She asked someone to call her husband, who drove her to the emergency room, where she waited 45 minutes while a man with a foot injury was treated first. When she was finally called into an exam room, an EKG revealed that she was having a heart attack. Doctors inserted a stent to restore blood flow to her heart and sent her home 5 days later with 11 prescriptions.

Another doctor referred her to the Heart Attack & Stroke Prevention Center in Spokane, Washington, where Bradley Bale, MD, diagnosed her with prediabetes, which boosts heart attack risk, as does the mutation in her KIF6 gene that genetic tests uncovered.

"Quite frankly, I consider the medical care she received to be substandard," says Dr. Bale. "If she'd been a man, no provider would have even considered an anxiety diagnosis without doing a full cardiac workup." As for her treatment in the ER? "If a man had come in with those symptoms, he would've gotten an immediate EKG, but the assumption was that this is just another hysterical female who is probably having a panic attack."

vessels—which is what happened to Niki. She now takes a blood thinner, a beta-blocker, and a statin, and she stopped working to focus on her health.

Screenings Niki should have had: advanced cholesterol test, carotid intimal medial thickness test (CIMT) (For more on these tests, see pages 219–220.)

CAMILLE KING

Camille, 47, is a credit manager in Peoria, Arizona.

When Camille felt light-headed and short of breath at work one day in July 2004, she chalked it up to stress. Her husband had just been laid off—3 days after they'd bought a new house.

Dr. Bale prescribed a statin, a beta-blocker, an ACE inhibitor, and a diabetes drug. A year later, after losing 45 pounds with a low-sugar diet and jogging, Camille no longer needed the diabetes drug. Her husband landed a job, too, lowering her financial stress. As for her own demanding position? She quit and found a new 8-hour-per-day job.

Screenings Camille should have had: advanced cholesterol test, stress echocardiography.

LAURA YOUNGER
Laura, 47, is an at-home mother in Gahanna, Ohio.

WILL YOUR INSURANCE PAY?

Compared with the $760,000 it costs to treat a single heart attack patient, these tests are cheap, but some insurers won't pay for them.

"The system rewards doctors who do bypasses but doesn't pay for prevention," says Arthur Agatston, MD, a preventive cardiologist and *Prevention* advisory board member.

Many companies are coming around: Most will pay for the stress EKG, A1c blood glucose, and advanced cholesterol tests. Some will cover the gene tests and CIMT. Cardiac calcium scoring usually isn't covered. Call your carrier beforehand to find out what it will pay for and what your copayment will be.

For a year, Laura couldn't shake her exhaustion. "I'd get out of breath walking up stairs," she says. Her doctor checked her twice for an underactive thyroid, which can also cause fatigue and shortness of breath, but said nothing was wrong.

At a football game in November 2006, Younger left the stands to go to the restroom. When she hadn't returned 20 minutes later, her husband found her sitting on the floor, out of breath, with neck and jaw pain—and without a single bystander offering to help. At the first-aid station, just after paramedics said her blood pressure was normal, she collapsed in full cardiac arrest.

An ambulance rushed her to Ohio State University Medical Center, where a catheterization revealed one of her arteries was 100 percent blocked and two were 85 percent clogged. She was put into a high-tech "cold suit" that chilled her body to 91°F, a treatment that reduces the brain's need for oxygen and helps it heal after a heart attack. Doctors then inserted stents to reopen the vessels.

When Laura woke up and found out what had happened, she had one thought: A heart attack? Me? Though overweight at 5 feet 7 inches and 175 pounds, she had no other risk factors that she knew of. She was referred to cardiac rehab, a 12- to 16-week recovery program increasingly being prescribed after heart attacks and paid for by insurance. Patients exercise under staff supervision and work with a nutritionist to

Seven Symptoms Women Ignore

Heart attack symptoms aren't unisex. "What we think of as characteristic heart attack pain—like an elephant sitting on your chest—is much more likely to occur in men than in women," says Marianne Legato, MD, director of the Partnership for Gender-Specific Medicine at Columbia University. In fact, 43 percent of women having a coronary don't experience any chest discomfort at all.

Women also wait longer to go to the ER than men do. (Their top reason for hesitating: They don't want to bother anyone.) But that can be fatal: Your odds of surviving improve by 23 percent if you get treatment within 3 hours and 50 percent if you get it within 1 hour.

Don't be a cardiac cautionary tale. If you have any of the following warning signs, act fast. As Dr. Legato says, "It's better to be embarrassed than dead."

Fatigue. In the weeks before an attack, 71 percent of women have flulike symptoms. Days before, you might feel too tired to lift your laptop.

Nonchest pain. Rather than an explosion in your chest, you may feel less severe pain in your upper back, shoulders, neck, or jaw.

Sweating. You might find yourself suddenly drenched in perspiration for no apparent reason, and your face may be pale or ashen.

Nausea or dizziness. During an attack, women often vomit or feel like they're going to pass out.

Breathlessness. Almost 58 percent of women report panting or an inability to carry on a conversation.

Sleeplessness. In the month before a coronary, nearly half of women have trouble sleeping.

Anxiety. "Many women experience a sense of impending doom or fear before a heart attack," says Dr. Legato. "That's your body telling you to pay attention. Trust those instincts."

improve their diets. But the day before she was to start, she was back in the ER with chest pain. This time the culprit was vaso- spasm, a sudden narrowing of an artery that chokes off blood flow to the heart. Surgeons implanted a defibrillator.

Laura sustained only minimal heart damage and was a star in rehab. "But when my mother died, I let my diet and exercise slide," she admits. She's back to her old weight.

However, the defibrillator has helped her stop living in fear. She takes six heart drugs, including a statin and a beta-blocker, has twice-yearly appointments with her cardiologist, and no longer sees the doctor who kept testing her thyroid.

Screenings Laura should have had: cardiac calcium scoring, CIMT.

Seven Tests You're Not Having That Could Save Your Life

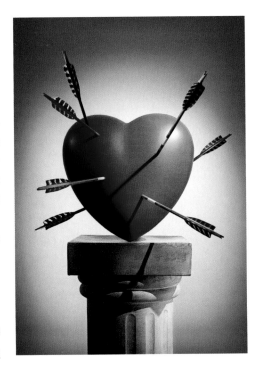

Think a stress test and a simple blood workup are all you need to assess your heart attack risk? Wrong.

If you haven't had these cutting-edge screenings, put this book down and call your doctor. Now.

Your physician has you come in to his office and run on a treadmill while you're hooked up to an EKG. For the next 8 to 12 minutes, he'll evaluate your heart rate, breathing, and blood pressure as the intensity of the workout increases. When the stress test is over, he'll tell you whether you have coronary artery disease.

Here's news that might make your heart skip a beat: For women, there's a 35 percent chance the test results will be wrong.

Most often, the test reveals false positives, meaning healthy women are told they have heart disease. Less frequently but obviously far more dangerous is when the test fails to detect clogged arteries that could, in fact, cause a heart attack. Fewer men are misdiagnosed.

A possible reason for the gender gap: Phases of the menstrual cycle and birth control pills have been shown to throw off results, indicating that estrogen's effects on heart cells might be a factor.

For decades, doctors had nothing more sophisticated than a stress test to offer. Not anymore. Cardiologists now use advanced imaging and blood tests that give a much more accurate assessment of heart attack risk.

"These tests are the best ways to tell who

is in danger, because they can catch cardio-vascular disease 20 to 30 years before it gets severe enough to cause a heart attack or stroke," says Arthur Agatston, MD, a preventive cardiologist and *Prevention* advisory board member, and an early champion of many of these tests.

Better detection is urgently needed: More than 1 million Americans have heart attacks every year and almost half die. Men have more than women do, but the gap is closing. From 1988 to 2004, attacks among women ages 35 to 54 spiked 42 percent.

These tests are available at most major medical centers and hospitals. If your doctor doesn't request them for you, demand the ones that are recommended for people in your age group and risk category.

Calcified plaque—a major warning sign of coronary artery disease, the leading cause of heart attacks—shows up at least 10 years before a heart attack or stroke hits. By catching the problem early, you can treat it before the buildup narrows arteries so severely that it triggers a heart attack.

Get it if. You're 50 or older with risk factors, or you're younger with a family history and several risk factors. Because the test involves x-rays, women shouldn't have it if there's any chance they might be pregnant.

Next steps. If your score is high, your doctor might advise lifestyle changes, a statin to lower your cholesterol, or a diabetes drug to lower blood sugar—all of which will also reduce plaque.

CARDIAC CALCIUM SCORING: CALCIUM IN THE CROSSHAIRS

How it works. A CT scanner checks for atherosclerotic plaque (made up of calcium, cholesterol, and scar tissue) in your heart's arteries. After electrodes are attached to your chest and to an EKG machine that monitors your heartbeat, you lie on an exam table that slides into a short, doughnut-shaped tunnel and hold your breath for 10 to 20 seconds.

Cost. $99 to $399

Duration. 10 minutes

Why it's heart smart. "Calcium scoring is the number one best predictor of a future heart attack," Dr. Agatston says.

CAROTID INTIMAL MEDIAL THICKNESS TEST: WHAT YOUR NECK KNOWS

How it works. This "ultrasound of the neck" takes a picture of the left and right carotid arteries, which supply blood to your head and brain. After putting a gel on your neck, a technician glides an ultrasound transducer over your carotids to measure the thickness of the arteries' lining.

Cost. $150 to $500

Duration. 15 minutes

Why it's heart smart. Studies show a link between abnormal thickness of the carotid lining and coronary artery disease.

"This test can detect even the earliest

stages, before blood flow is blocked," says Dr. Agatston. Because it's not an x-ray, it's also helpful for women who are or may be pregnant.

Get it if. You're 40 or older, or you're under 40 and a close relative (parents or siblings) had a heart attack or stroke before age 55.

Next steps. A diet and exercise plan, stress reduction, and, if necessary, drugs to lower your cholesterol, blood pressure, and blood sugar, and reduce your intimal medial thickness.

HIGH-SENSITIVITY C-REACTIVE PROTEIN TEST: INFLAMMATION FINDER

How it works. A blood test measures CRP, a protein in your blood that's a strong indicator of inflammation throughout your body.

Cost. $8

Duration. 5 minutes

Why it's heart smart. Cholesterol plaque injures blood vessels, triggering inflammation and raising CRP levels in your blood. That's dangerous because women with high levels of CRP may be up to four times more likely to suffer a heart attack or stroke. A high CRP is most dangerous if you also have another risk factor: a waist circumference of more than 35 inches, indicating the presence of belly fat.

Get it if. You're 40 or older.

Next steps. A statin, along with weight loss and exercise, can cut risk of heart problems in people with high CRP.

ADVANCED LIPID PROFILE AND LIPOPROTEIN(A) TEST: CHOLESTEROL COUNTERS

How they work. Unlike the traditional cholesterol blood test, which measures total cholesterol, HDL, LDL, and triglycerides, the advanced test also looks at particle size. This is important because some particles are big and fluffy, so they tend to bounce off artery walls as they travel through the body. Others are small and dense, meaning they can penetrate the artery lining and form clumps of plaque. (Think beach balls versus bullets.) The Lp(a) blood test analyzes a specific type of cholesterol that can triple heart risk.

Cost. $19 each

Duration. 5 minutes

Why they're heart smart. Sizing up your particles gives a clearer picture of heart risk than the conventional test: Having a lot of large particles cuts risk, while small ones raise it. The more Lp(a) you have, the worse it is, too; it makes LDL particles extra sticky, so they cling to the lining of blood vessels, causing plaque and clots.

Get them if. You have a family history of heart disease.

Next steps. If you have small particles, your doctor may prescribe a drug to increase their size, most likely a fenofibrate (such as TriCor or Trilipix) or niacin (vitamin B_3), along with a healthy diet and exercise. Niacin is also the best treatment for high Lp(a).

A1C BLOOD GLUCOSE TEST: SORTING OUT SUGAR

How it works. If you have diabetes, you're probably very familiar with this test. A blood test indicates your average level of blood sugar over the prior 3 months. Unlike other glucose tests that require fasting or drinking a sugary beverage, this test requires neither.

Cost. $50

Duration. 5 minutes

Why it's heart smart. "This is the simplest way to detect your future risk of diabetes," Dr. Agatston says. This disease puts you at five times higher risk of developing heart disease, yet 5.7 million Americans have undiagnosed diabetes (on top of the 17.9 million who are diagnosed) because they haven't had their blood sugar checked.

Get it if. You're 45 or older, or earlier if you're overweight and have one or more diabetes risk factors, such as family history, high triglycerides, or low HDL.

Next steps. Diabetes can often be reversed with weight loss, exercise, and dietary changes, such as the many recommended in this book. If that's not enough, you may need oral medication or insulin injections.

GENETIC TESTS: DNA DETECTION

How they work. A blood sample is tested at a lab for mutations of the KIF6 and APOE genes.

Cost. $130 each

Duration. 5 minutes

Why they're heart smart. A common variation in the KIF6 gene and two mutations in the APOE gene raise your heart disease risk. "You have no control over your genes," says Dr. Agatston, "but these tests can help your doctor better tailor your treatment to head off a heart attack."

Get them if. You're 40 or older.

Next steps. A drug to lower cholesterol, changes in diet, or both.

THINK YOU'RE HAVING A HEART ATTACK? TAKE THESE THREE STEPS

Call 911. Don't drive yourself to the ER, and don't ask someone else to take you. In the ambulance, treatment can begin right away, and they can speed you to the nearest medical center that can handle acute cardiac arrest.

Take an aspirin. Keep a supply of full-strength uncoated aspirin at home and in your purse, and chew and swallow one with water as soon as symptoms start. This can help prevent blood clotting and the damage it causes.

Get pushy at the ER. Or ask a relative or friend to be your advocate. Forcefully say, "I think I'm having a heart attack," and insist on seeing a doctor within 10 minutes. Make sure you get an EKG to check your heart function, and blood tests to detect heart damage. Do not leave the hospital until you've been evaluated by a cardiologist.

STRESS ECHOCARDIOGRAPHY: A SUPER STRESS TEST

How it works. This test is an improvement over the standard stress test because it adds an ultrasound both before and after exercise to evaluate blood flow to your heart's pumping chambers and to check for blockages in the arteries that supply the heart.

Cost. $850 to $1,600

Duration. 45 minutes

Why it's heart smart. Adding echocardiography to the standard stress test raises accuracy by as much as 85 percent for women.

"It's an excellent way to tell if your heart disease is severe enough that you could require treatments like a stent or a bypass," Dr. Agatston says.

Get it if. You have signs of heart disease, regardless of your age. "If you experience shortness of breath, chest pain, neck pain, or any other symptom, you need this test," he says. (See "Seven Symptoms Women Ignore" on page 217.)

Next steps. Your doctor may recommend a cardiac catheterization to check for blockages. If your vessels are clogged, they can be reopened with angioplasty, a stent, or bypass surgery.

ASSESS YOUR HEART DISEASE RISK

You're at risk if you smoke; load up on saturated fats; don't exercise; or have high blood pressure, high cholesterol, diabetes, or a family history of heart disease. But the following habits and hazards are also dangerous.

Psoriasis. Because it triggers inflammation inside the body, this chronic skin disease boosts your chances of cardiovascular disease nearly as much as smoking does.

Skimping on sleep. Getting 5 or fewer hours a night more than doubles the danger, even in otherwise healthy people.

Gum disease. People who have periodontal disease—bacterial infection of the gums—are nearly twice as likely to have a fatal heart attack as those who don't. Almost 75 percent of adults have unhealthy gums, many without realizing it, because oral infection is painless in the early stages.

Pregnancy complication. For women, having preeclampsia (high blood pressure and protein in the urine) doubles the odds of a heart attack later in life; developing gestational diabetes ups this risk by 70 percent.

Workplace stress. People with demanding jobs but little control over how to perform them have a 40 percent higher risk of heart attack and stroke than those with low-stress jobs. Job insecurity is linked to high blood pressure, high cholesterol, and weight gain, all of which take a toll on heart health.

The Truth about Statins

If you walk into your doctor's office with high cholesterol, you might, like 30 million other Americans, walk out with a prescription for a statin—a drug such as Lipitor, Crestor, or Zocor. Statins, which block a liver enzyme that helps create cholesterol, work wonders for some: The average person taking one will see her bad LDL drop between 20 and 60 percent in a month. Little wonder that statins have become this country's most widely prescribed drug.

"These medications are highly effective for lowering cholesterol, which can reduce risk of a heart attack," says Steven Nissen, MD, chair of the Cleveland Clinic's department of cardiovascular medicine and a *Prevention* advisory board member.

Statins achieve this with relatively few side effects. Even the serious ones—muscle pain, numbness, and memory problems, experienced by 5 to 10 percent of statin patients—stop within a few days or weeks after the person is taken off the drug. What's less understood by the public, though, is that a statin is not an inoculation against a heart attack.

"If you think a statin alone will protect you, you're absolutely wrong," says Arthur Agatston, MD, a preventive cardiologist and *Prevention* advisory board member.

How can that be? For one thing, it takes a lot more than good cholesterol numbers to prevent a heart attack. "Even if a statin lowers your LDL, heart disease can still develop," says Dr. Agatston, explaining that several other factors, from genetics to lifestyle, also affect cardiac health.

In addition, approximately 7 million Americans taking statins don't need their LDL lowered to begin with. They have normal cholesterol levels but are given a statin because they have other risk factors. The prevailing wisdom is that a statin might provide extra insurance against a heart attack.

A recent 6-year study looked at 2,100 adults who had normal cholesterol levels but were being considered for statin therapy. The results showed that only those with significant calcium buildup in their arteries—a sign that heart disease was already in progress—could be expected to benefit from the drug.

The jury has been out as to whether statins benefit women as much as they help men, because most studies have been done only on men. A March 2010 study, however, shows that at least one statin does quantifiably benefit women. Researchers at Brigham and Women's Hospital analyzed data from 6,800 women and found that they experienced a 46 percent drop in "cardiovascular events" (including bypass surgery and hospitalization for chest pain), a slight edge over the 42 percent decline for men.

The bottom line is that women should insist on a thorough, tailored medical assessment.

BREAKFASTS

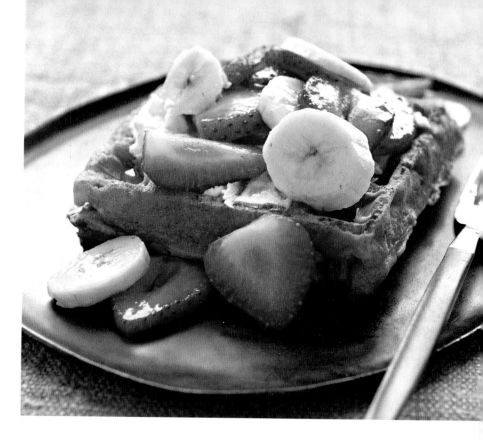

PEANUT BUTTER WAFFLE
WITH BANANA AND STRAWBERRIES

MAKES 1 SERVING

- 1 frozen whole wheat waffle, toasted
- 2 tablespoons natural peanut butter
- 1 tablespoon ricotta cheese
- ½ small banana, sliced
- 3 strawberries, sliced

Spread the waffle with the peanut butter and ricotta. Top with the banana and strawberry slices.

PER SERVING:
380 CAL

12 g protein
37 g carbohydrates
21 g fat
4 g saturated fat
6 g fiber
344 mg sodium

DOUBLE PUMPKIN SNACK BARS

MAKES 12 SERVINGS

1½ cups shelled pumpkin seeds

1 cup canned solid-pack pumpkin

1 large carrot, shredded (about 1 cup)

½ cup sugar

⅓ cup dried cranberries or raisins, chopped

¼ cup canola oil

2 eggs

1 cup whole grain pastry flour

1 teaspoon baking powder

1 teaspoon ground cinnamon

½ teaspoon baking soda

¼ teaspoon salt

1. Preheat the oven to 350°F. Coat a 13″ × 9″ × 2″ baking pan with cooking spray.
2. Measure 1 cup of the pumpkin seeds into a blender or food processor and process until finely ground. Set aside. Coarsely chop the remaining seeds and set aside.
3. In a large bowl, combine the pumpkin, carrot, sugar, cranberries or raisins, oil, and eggs and stir until well blended. Add the flour, ground pumpkin seeds, baking powder, cinnamon, baking soda, and salt. Mix until blended.
4. Pour the batter into the prepared pan and spread evenly. Sprinkle with the reserved chopped pumpkin seeds. Bake for 22 to 25 minutes, or until the top springs back when pressed lightly. Cool completely in the pan on a rack before cutting into 12 bars.

STRAWBERRY-ALMOND-TOPPED FRENCH TOAST

MAKES 1 SERVING

- 1 egg
- ¼ cup fat-free milk
- ¼ teaspoon ground cinnamon
- 1 slice whole grain bread
- 1 teaspoon trans-free margarine
- ½ cup sliced strawberries
- 2 tablespoons sliced almonds, toasted

PER SERVING:

304 CAL

16 g protein	
26 g carbohydrates	
16 g fat	
3 g saturated fat	
5 g fiber	
270 mg sodium	

1. In a shallow bowl, beat the egg with the milk and cinnamon. Dip both sides of the bread in the egg mixture.
2. In a nonstick skillet over medium heat, melt the margarine. Cook the bread for about 2 to 3 minutes per side, or until golden. Cut in half diagonally. Place half on a plate. Top with half of the strawberries and almonds. Cover with the other toast half and the remaining strawberries and almonds.

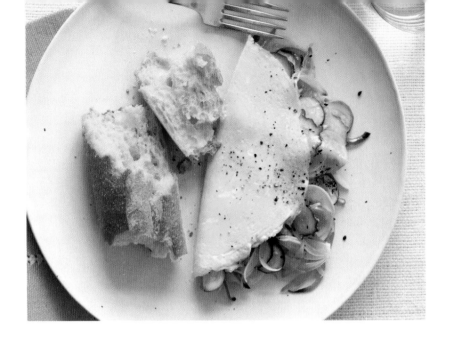

CLASSIC CHEESE OMELET

PER SERVING:

296 CAL

17 g protein
5 g carbohydrates
24 g fat
7 g saturated fat
1 g fiber
377 mg sodium

MAKES 1 SERVING

- 2 eggs
- 1 teaspoon water
- Pinch of salt
- Pinch of freshly ground black pepper
- 2 teaspoons olive oil, divided
- ¼ cup thinly sliced red onion
- ¼ cup sliced zucchini and/or yellow squash
- 2 tablespoons grated Cheddar cheese

1. In a medium bowl, beat the eggs, water, salt, and pepper just to blend.
2. In an 8" nonstick skillet, heat 1 teaspoon of the oil over medium-high heat. Cook the onion, zucchini, and/or squash, stirring occasionally, for 5 minutes. Remove to a plate. In the same skillet, heat the remaining 1 teaspoon oil over medium heat. Pour in the egg mixture. Stir constantly with a heat-proof rubber spatula until the eggs thicken to a custardy consistency, for 10 to 20 seconds.
3. Tilt the pan to allow any uncooked egg to run to the side. Run the spatula all around the edge of the omelet.
4. Sprinkle the cheese over half of the omelet. Top with the onion mixture. Fold the other half over the top. Turn off the heat and let stand for 30 seconds to set around the filling. Gently push the omelet onto a plate with the spatula. Sprinkle with additional pepper, if desired.

SPINACH FRITTATA

MAKES 4 SERVINGS

- 4 eggs
- 4 egg whites
- ¼ cup grated Asiago cheese
- ¼ teaspoon salt
- 1 small onion, finely chopped
- 1 red bell pepper, cut into thin strips
- ¼ cup finely chopped Canadian bacon
- 4 cups fresh baby spinach

PER SERVING:
149 CAL

14 g protein	
7 g carbohydrates	
7 g fat	
3 g saturated fat	
2 g fiber	
492 mg sodium	

1. Preheat the oven to 350°F.
2. In a medium bowl, whisk together the eggs, egg whites, cheese, and salt.
3. Coat a large, ovenproof, nonstick skillet with cooking spray and heat over medium heat. Add the onion, pepper, and bacon and cook for 4 minutes, or until browned. Add the spinach and cook, stirring, for 1 minute, or until the spinach is wilted. Pour in the egg mixture and cook for 2 minutes, or until the bottom of the frittata is starting to set.
4. Place in the oven and bake for 10 minutes, or until set.

HERBED BREAKFAST SCRAMBLE

MAKES 4 SERVINGS

2 tablespoons canola oil

1 small red onion, finely chopped

1 container (14 ounces) soft tofu packed in calcium sulfate, drained

¼ teaspoon salt

⅛ teaspoon freshly ground black pepper

⅛ teaspoon turmeric

1 cup shredded reduced-fat Cheddar cheese

2 tablespoons chopped fresh basil

1 tablespoon chopped fresh thyme

1. In a large skillet, heat the oil over medium heat. Cook the onion for 5 minutes, or until tender. Crumble the tofu into the pan. Sprinkle with the salt, pepper, and turmeric. Cook for 5 minutes, stirring frequently, until firm and lightly browned.

2. Remove the skillet from the heat. Add the cheese, basil, and thyme and stir until the cheese melts.

BREAKFAST BURRITOS

MAKES 6 SERVINGS

PER SERVING:

161 CAL

11 g protein	
16 g carbohydrates	
6 g fat	
2.5 g saturated fat	
3 g fiber	
531 mg sodium	

1 package (14 ounces) light tofu packed in calcium sulfate (we used Nasoya)

3 omega-3-enhanced whole wheat tortillas (8" diameter)

1 red bell pepper, chopped

1 small onion, chopped

1/4 teaspoon ground cumin

1/2 cup salsa

1/4 cup fresh cilantro

1 cup (4 ounces) shredded reduced-fat Cheddar cheese

3 cups fresh baby spinach

1. Preheat the oven to 350°F.
2. Remove the tofu from the package and place it in a colander in the sink. Place a flat plate on top of the tofu and a heavy can of vegetables on the plate for 5 minutes to drain.
3. Wrap the tortillas in foil and place them in the oven to heat.
4. Coat a large nonstick skillet with cooking spray and heat over medium heat. Cook the pepper, onion, and cumin for 5 minutes, or until tender. Crumble the tofu into the pan and cook for 2 minutes, or until lightly browned. Add the salsa and cilantro and cook for 5 minutes, stirring frequently, or until heated through. Top with the cheese and cook for 2 minutes to melt.
5. Lay 1 tortilla on a flat surface. Top with 1/2 cup of the spinach and approximately 1/2 cup of the tofu mixture. Roll to seal, then cut in half. Repeat with the remaining tortillas, spinach, and tofu mixture.

SOUTHERN SHRIMP AND GRITS

PER SERVING:
262 CAL

26 g protein

25 g
carbohydrates

6 g fat

1 g
saturated fat

1 g fiber

417 mg sodium

MAKES 4 SERVINGS

2 cups fat-free milk

2 tablespoons nonfat dry milk

½ cup dry white grits

¼ cup grated Parmesan cheese

2 teaspoons canola oil

¾ pound medium shrimp, peeled

4 scallions, sliced

1 teaspoon Cajun seasoning

1. In a saucepan, combine the milk and dry milk. Bring to a simmer over medium heat. Whisk in the grits. Bring the mixture just to a boil, stirring occasionally. Cover partially and reduce the heat. Simmer, stirring occasionally, for 12 to 15 minutes, or until very thick. Remove the saucepan from the heat. Stir in the cheese.
2. Heat a nonstick skillet over medium-high heat. Add the oil and swirl to coat the pan. Add the shrimp, scallions, and Cajun seasoning. Toss for 5 minutes, or until the shrimp are opaque.
3. Divide the grits among 4 plates. Top with the shrimp mixture.

PEANUT-OATS BREAKFAST PUDDING

MAKES 1 SERVING

- ¼ cup nonfat dry milk
- 1½ tablespoons natural reduced-fat peanut butter
- ½ cup water
- ¼ cup rolled oats
- 1 tablespoon fat-free plain yogurt
- 1 teaspoon finely chopped peanuts

1. In a 4-cup microwaveable bowl or mixing cup, whisk 2 tablespoons of the dry milk with the peanut butter until creamy. While whisking, gradually add the water and the remaining dry milk and whisk until the mixture is smooth. Stir in the oats.

2. Cover the bowl with plastic wrap, leaving a small vent for steam to escape. Microwave on high power for 1 minute. Reduce the power to medium and cook for about 90 seconds, or until creamy. Remove and allow to sit for 5 minutes.

3. Spoon the mixture into a cereal bowl and top with the yogurt and peanuts.

APPETIZERS AND SNACKS

WALNUT–GOAT CHEESE DIP

MAKES 6 SERVINGS

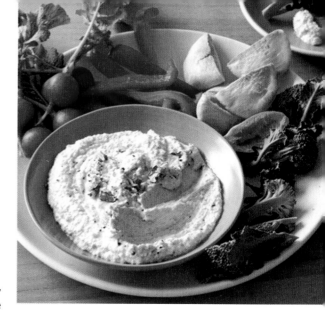

- 1/3 cup walnut pieces
- 1 1/2 tablespoons water
- 1 tablespoon vodka
- 1 tablespoon chopped scallion (white part only)
- 1/8 teaspoon freshly ground black pepper
- 4 ounces soft goat cheese, at room temperature

In a food processor, combine the walnuts, water, vodka, scallion, and pepper and pulse until the nuts are finely chopped and a smooth paste forms, scraping down the sides as needed. Add the cheese and process until well blended.

PER SERVING:
100 CAL

5 g protein	
1 g carbohydrates	
8 g fat	
3 g saturated fat	
1 g fiber	
70 mg sodium	

Superfood: Walnuts

Nuts give sweet or savory dishes flavor, crunch, and a heart-healthy punch. Even better? Walnuts score highest of all nuts in the omega-3s that protect against heart disease. Just three walnuts a day supply your daily goal for omega-3 fats. Their stores of fiber and unsaturated fat can help you lower "bad" LDL cholesterol naturally.

To preserve taste and prevent spoiling, keep shelled nuts refrigerated in an airtight container for up to 6 months or in the freezer for up to a year.

HERBED CHEESE BALL WITH CRUDITÉS

MAKES 8 SERVINGS

- 6 ounces Neufchâtel
- ¾ cup shredded reduced-fat, extra-sharp Cheddar cheese
- 1 tablespoon prepared horseradish
- 2 teaspoons Worcestershire sauce
- ¼ cup walnuts, very finely chopped
- 16 fat-free plain rice cakes
- 4 ribs celery, cut into 2"-long pieces
- 4 carrots, cut into sticks
- 1 large cucumber, diagonally cut into ¼"-thick slices

1. In a blender or food processor, combine the Neufchâtel, Cheddar, horseradish, and Worcestershire sauce. Pulse until just blended. Place in a bowl and refrigerate for at least 1 hour. Remove and shape into a ball.
2. Place the walnuts on a plate and roll the cheese ball in the nuts, pressing to adhere.
3. Place the cheese ball on a serving plate with a canapé knife and surround with the rice cakes, celery, carrots, and cucumber.

SPICY SNACK MIX

MAKES 18 SERVINGS (½ CUP PER SERVING)

- ½ cup canola oil
- 1 tablespoon chili powder
- 1 teaspoon ground cumin
- 1 teaspoon dried oregano
- ½ teaspoon salt
- ¼ teaspoon ground red pepper
- 3 cups multigrain cereal squares
- 2¼ cups unsalted sunflower seeds
- 2 cups oat or multigrain cereal
- 2 cups multigrain pretzel sticks

PER SERVING
230 CAL

5 g protein
22 g carbohydrates
15 g fat
1.5 g saturated fat
3 g fiber
320 mg sodium

1. In a small measuring cup, combine the oil, chili powder, cumin, oregano, salt, and pepper.
2. In a 3½- to 5-quart slow cooker, combine the cereal squares, sunflower seeds, cereal, and pretzels. Drizzle with the oil mixture, tossing to coat well. Cover and cook on low for 2 to 3 hours, stirring twice during the cooking time. Be sure to check the mixture after 2 hours, because slow cooker times can vary.
3. Remove the lid during the last half hour of cooking to allow the mix to dry.

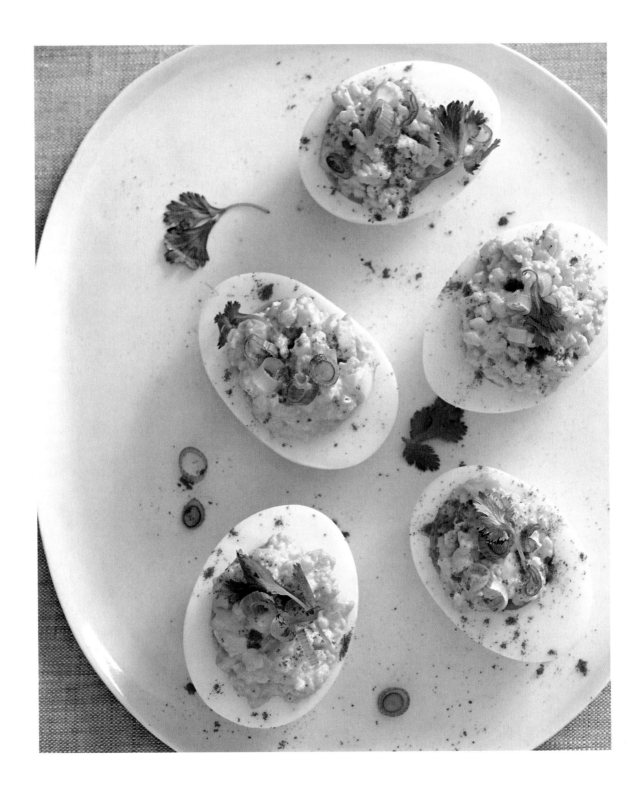

MEXICANA DEVILED EGGS

MAKES 8 SERVINGS

- 6 hard-cooked eggs
- 2 tablespoons mayonnaise
- ¼ teaspoon chili powder + additional for garnish
- 1 scallion, finely sliced
- 1 tablespoon chopped fresh cilantro

1. Shell the eggs. Place 2 eggs in a shallow bowl. Cut the remaining 4 eggs into halves lengthwise. Remove the yolks and add them to the eggs in the bowl. With a fork or pastry blender, mash the eggs and yolks in the bowl. Add the mayonnaise and ¼ teaspoon chili powder. Stir to mix.

2. Place the egg white halves on a plate, hollow side up. Dollop the yolk mixture into the hollows. Scatter the scallion and cilantro on top. Dust the plate with the additional chili powder.

PER SERVING:
69 CAL

5 g protein	
2 g carbohydrates	
4 g fat	
1 g saturated fat	
0 g fiber	
84 mg sodium	

ANTIPASTO PIZZA

MAKES 6 SERVINGS

    3 tablespoons prepared sun-dried tomato pesto
  12" thin-crust pizza shell (we used Boboli)
    3 ounces shredded provolone cheese (about 1 cup)
    3 ounces jarred roasted red peppers, thinly sliced
    6 ounces marinated artichoke hearts, drained and roughly chopped
    5 pitted and halved kalamata olives
    3 slices salami, cut into strips

1. Preheat the oven to 450°F.
2. Spread the pesto over the pizza crust, leaving a ½" border. Top with the cheese, red peppers, artichoke hearts, and olives. Bake on the top rack until the crust is crisp, for about 10 minutes. Remove the pizza from the oven. Scatter the salami on top. Cut into 8 wedges.

TIME-SAVERS

Preheat the oven or put a pot of water on to boil as soon as you walk in the door. You'll be minutes closer to dinner. Take a shortcut to healthy ingredients. Rotisserie chicken? Precut vegetables? Prewashed greens? Bring 'em on, and let them jump-start a good-for-you meal. When you need a small quantity, hit the salad bar for ready-prepped ingredients. Buy just what you need—no waste! Keep your pantry, refrigerator, and freezer stocked with quick-cook staples. If you already have ingredients such as canned beans, stock, and tuna; dried pasta and grains; jarred and bottled sauces; grated cheese; and frozen vegetable blends, you won't even need to stop at the market.

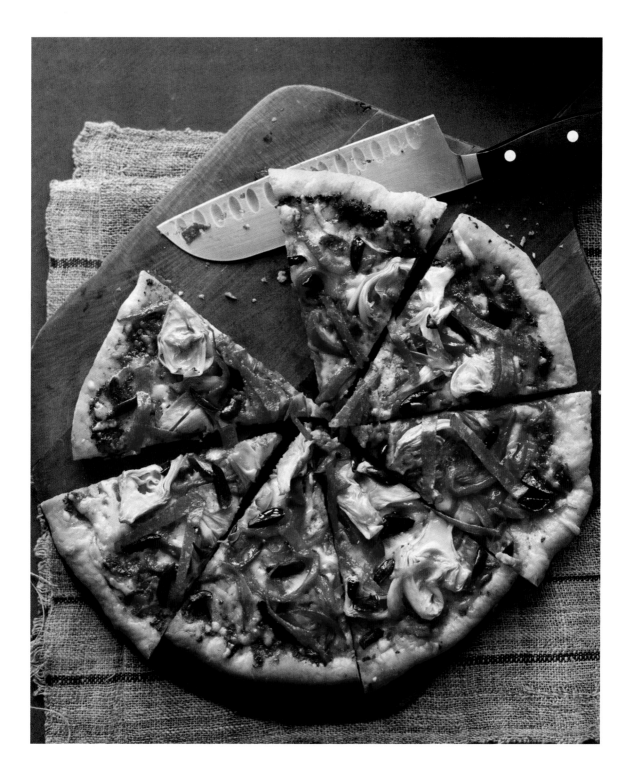

SAVORY ARTICHOKE-TOMATO TART

PER SERVING:

128 CAL

12 g protein
7 g carbohydrates
5 g fat
1 g saturated fat
1 g fiber
301 mg sodium

MAKES 10 SERVINGS

- 3 tablespoons ground flaxseed
- 1 tablespoon canola oil
- 6 canned artichokes, rinsed, drained, and quartered
- 1/2 cup sliced grape tomatoes
- 2 cups reduced-fat ricotta cheese
- 3 eggs, beaten
- 1/4 cup grated Romano cheese
- 2 tablespoons chopped parsley
- 1 tablespoon cornstarch
- 1/2 teaspoon dried oregano
- 1/2 teaspoon freshly ground black pepper
- 1/4 teaspoon salt

1. Position an oven rack in the bottom third of the oven. Preheat the oven to 325°F. Coat the bottom and sides of an 8″ springform pan with cooking spray.
2. In a small bowl, combine the flaxseed and oil with a fork. Sprinkle the mixture evenly over the pan bottom. (There may be some bare patches.) Set aside.
3. Place the artichokes and tomatoes, cut side down, on several layers of paper towels. Pat dry with paper towels.
4. In a mixing bowl, whisk the ricotta until smooth. Gradually add the eggs, whisking until smooth. Add the cheese, parsley, cornstarch, oregano, pepper, and salt. Whisk just until combined. Dollop the mixture into the prepared pan. Spread to smooth. Place the artichokes and tomatoes, cut side up, on top. Press with the back of a spatula to embed the vegetables.
5. Bake for about 35 minutes, or until set. Remove and allow to cool for at least 1 hour before serving. Or, cover and refrigerate for up to 24 hours.
6. To serve, cut into 10 slices.

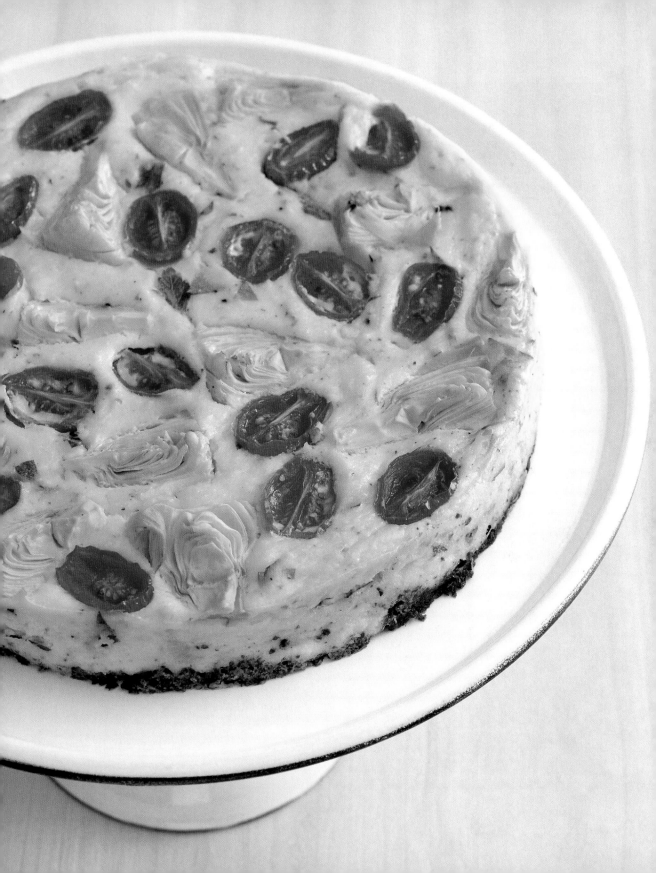

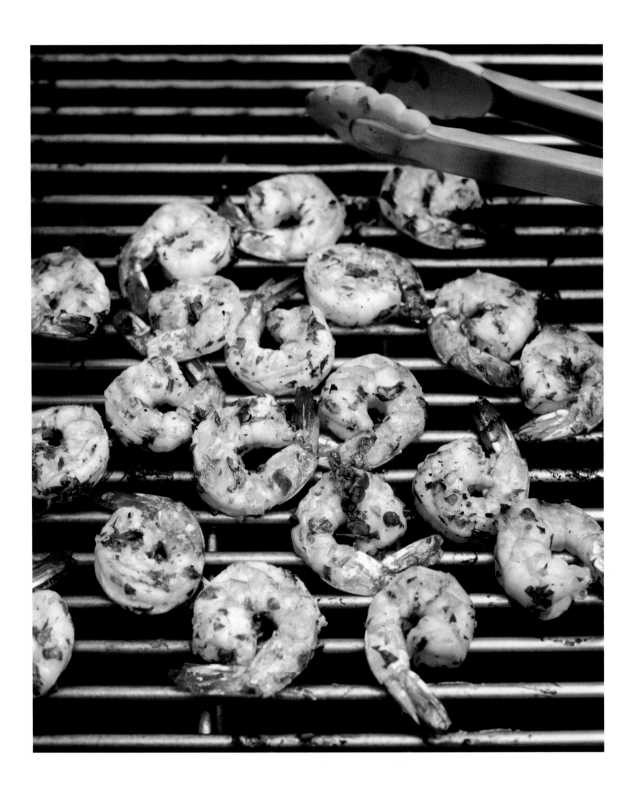

LEMON-PEPPER SHRIMP

MAKES 4 SERVINGS

1 pound extra-large shrimp (16–20 count), peeled

2 tablespoons extra virgin olive oil

2 large cloves garlic, crushed or put through garlic press

2 teaspoons freshly grated lemon zest

½ teaspoon freshly ground black pepper

¼ teaspoon red-pepper flakes

¼ cup + 2 teaspoons freshly squeezed lemon juice (from 2 lemons)

2 tablespoons finely chopped parsley

2 tablespoons + 2 teaspoons dry white wine

2 tablespoons butter

2 tablespoons drained capers, chopped (optional)

Salt and ground black pepper

Lemon wedges (optional)

PER SERVING:
251 CAL

23 g protein

4 g carbohydrates

15 g fat

5 g saturated fat

1 g fiber

211 mg sodium

1. In a medium bowl, place the shrimp, oil, garlic, lemon zest, black pepper, and red-pepper flakes. Add ¼ cup of the lemon juice and 1 tablespoon of the parsley. Marinate for 15 to 30 minutes.
2. Coat a grill rack with cooking spray. Heat the grill to medium.
3. Place the wine, butter, 2 teaspoons lemon juice, and capers (if using) in a saucepan over high heat. Bring to a boil and remove from the heat.
4. Put the shrimp on the grill and sprinkle with salt and pepper. Grill until bright pink, about 2 minutes per side. Transfer to a bowl and stir in the warm butter mixture. Sprinkle with 1 tablespoon of the parsley. Garnish with the lemon wedges (if using).

ASIAN SALMON BITES

PER SERVING:

191 CAL

13 g protein

14 g
carbohydrates

10 g fat

2 g
saturated fat

3 g fiber

478 mg sodium

MAKES 4 SERVINGS (5 BITES PER SERVING)

1 pouch (6 ounces) salmon, patted dry

⅓ cup dried bread crumbs

1 carrot, shredded

2 scallions, finely chopped

1 tablespoon reduced-sodium soy sauce

2 teaspoons finely grated fresh ginger

4 tablespoons fat-free Greek yogurt

⅓ cup sesame seeds

1 teaspoon wasabi paste

¼ cup drained pickled ginger

1. In a medium bowl, combine the salmon, bread crumbs, carrot, scallions, soy sauce, ginger, and 2 tablespoons of the yogurt, ¼ cup of the sesame seeds, and ½ teaspoon of the wasabi paste. Stir until well blended. Chill.

2. Stir together the remaining 2 tablespoons of yogurt and ½ teaspoon of wasabi paste until combined. Chill.

3. Preheat the oven to 400°F. Coat a baking sheet with cooking spray.

4. Place the remaining sesame seeds on a plate. Form 1 tablespoon of the salmon mixture into a patty and repeat, making 20 patties. Working one at a time, press into the sesame seeds to coat.

5. Place the patties on the prepared baking sheet. Spray the tops of the patties with cooking spray. Bake for 10 to 12 minutes, turning twice, or until browned.

6. Place the salmon bites on a serving plate. Top each with a generous teaspoon of the yogurt mixture and a small piece of the pickled ginger. Sprinkle with any remaining sesame seeds.

MUSSELS ROCKEFELLER

MAKES 4 SERVINGS (6 MUSSELS PER SERVING)

24	mussels, scrubbed (about 1 pound)
3	cups fresh baby spinach
1	clove garlic, finely chopped
	Pinch of salt
1½	teaspoons ground flaxseed
	Hot-pepper sauce
2	tablespoons grated Parmesan cheese

13 g protein

6 g
carbohydrates

3 g fat

1 g
saturated fat

1 g fiber

427 mg sodium

1. Preheat the broiler. Set out a 13″ × 9″ baking dish.
2. Place the mussels in a large nonstick skillet. Cover and set over high heat. Cook, tossing occasionally, for 2 to 3 minutes, or until the shells open. Discard any shells that don't open. With tongs, remove the mussels one at a time, tipping the shells to drain any juices into the pan. Set the mussels on a tray.
3. Add the spinach, garlic, and salt to the pan. Cover and set over medium-high heat. Cook for 2 minutes, or until wilted. Add the flaxseed and a couple of dashes of hot-pepper sauce. Stir with a fork to blend.
4. Remove and discard the empty shell half of each mussel. Place the shell halves with the mussel attached in the baking dish. Spoon some of the spinach mixture on each mussel. Sprinkle with the cheese.
5. Broil 6″ from the heat for about 2 minutes, or until bubbling.

ROASTED ASPARAGUS SPEARS WITH MUSTARD SAUCE

PER SERVING:

68 CAL

8 g protein
6 g carbohydrates
2 g fat
0.5 g saturated fat
2 g fiber
128 mg sodium

MAKES 4 SERVINGS (5 SPEARS WITH MUSTARD SAUCE PER SERVING)

20 spears asparagus, trimmed if necessary

1 teaspoon canola oil

½ cup reduced-fat ricotta cheese

2 tablespoons nonfat dry milk

2 tablespoons grated Parmesan cheese

2 teaspoons whole grain mustard

1 teaspoon prepared horseradish

1. Preheat the oven to 425°F.
2. Place the asparagus on a baking sheet (with sides) large enough to hold them in a single layer. Drizzle with the oil and toss to coat the spears.
3. Bake for 15 to 17 minutes, or until the asparagus is crisp-tender. (Baking time will vary, depending upon thickness.)
4. Meanwhile, in a bowl, combine the ricotta, dry milk, Parmesan, mustard, and horseradish.
5. Place 5 asparagus spears on each of 4 appetizer plates. Dollop the sauce on the spears.

PEA PODS WITH FETA-HERB FILLING

MAKES 10 SERVINGS (3 PODS PER SERVING)

- ½ cup reduced-fat ricotta cheese
- ½ cup reduced-fat feta cheese
- 1½ tablespoons finely chopped fresh dill
- ½ teaspoon grated orange zest
  Coarsely ground black pepper
- 30 snow peas
- 1 tablespoon finely chopped walnuts

1. In a medium bowl, combine the ricotta, feta, dill, and orange zest. Season liberally with the pepper. Mash with a fork to combine.

2. Slit open the straighter side of the pea pods with a small, sharp knife. Fill each pod with some of the cheese mixture, using a small spoon or knife. Place on a serving plate, sitting each pod upright like a rowboat. Sprinkle the walnuts over the pea pods.

TUNA SALAD ON BED OF GREENS

PER SERVING:

305 CAL

28 g protein	
23 g carbohydrates	
11 g fat	
3 g saturated fat	
5 g fiber	
388 mg sodium	

MAKES 2 SERVINGS

- 2 slices whole grain bread, cut into 1" cubes
- ¼ cup low-fat plain yogurt
- 1 tablespoon mayonnaise
- 1 tablespoon lemon juice
- ¼ teaspoon lemon zest
- 1 can (6 ounces) low-sodium waterpacked white tuna, drained
- ¼ small red onion, finely chopped
- 2 tablespoons chopped parsley leaves
- 2 teaspoons capers, rinsed, drained, and chopped
- 3 cups mesclun or spring mix
- 1 large carrot, peeled into long strips
- 1 tomato, halved lengthwise and sliced

1. Preheat the oven to 400°F.
2. Place the cubes on a baking sheet with sides and coat with canola cooking spray. Toss to coat all sides of the cubes. Bake for 5 minutes or until toasted, tossing once. Set aside.
3. In a large bowl, stir together the yogurt, mayonnaise, lemon juice, and lemon zest. Add the tuna, onion, parsley, and capers.
4. Divide the mesclun, carrot, and tomato between 2 plates. Top with the tuna mixture. Sprinkle with the croutons.

CITRUS-ARUGULA SALAD WITH GRILLED CHICKEN

MAKES 4 SERVINGS

¼ cup orange juice

2 tablespoons lemon juice

2 tablespoons lime juice

1 tablespoon honey

3 cloves garlic, minced

1 teaspoon dried thyme

4 boneless, skinless chicken breast halves (4 ounces each)

2 tablespoons canola oil

½ cup fat-free Greek yogurt

8 cups arugula

2 beets, peeled and shredded

PER SERVING:

262 CAL

27 g protein

16 g carbohydrates

10 g fat

1 g saturated fat

2 g fiber

192 mg sodium

1. In a shallow covered dish, whisk together the orange juice, lemon juice, lime juice, honey, garlic, and thyme. Add the chicken, turning to coat. Cover and refrigerate for 1 to 2 hours, turning occasionally. (The chicken can marinate for up to 12 hours, if desired.)
2. Coat a broiler pan or grill rack with cooking spray. Preheat the broiler or grill.
3. Place the chicken on the broiler pan or grill rack, reserving the marinade. Cook for 15 minutes, or until a thermometer inserted in the thickest portion registers 160°F and the juices run clear.
4. Meanwhile, in a small saucepan, place the marinade over high heat. Bring to a boil and boil for 3 minutes. Remove from the heat and whisk in the oil. Gently whisk in the yogurt.
5. Divide the arugula and beets among 4 plates. Slice the chicken, place it on the salads, and drizzle with the marinade.

EASY EGG SALAD PLATTER

PER SERVING:

277 CAL

13 g protein

22 g
carbohydrates

16 g fat

2 g
saturated fat

5 g fiber

400 mg sodium

MAKES 4 SERVINGS

6 hard-cooked eggs, peeled (discard 3 yolks)

3 ribs celery, chopped

½ cup peeled, chopped cucumber

3 radishes, chopped

2 scallions, thinly sliced, or ¼ cup chopped sweet white onion

¼ cup mayonnaise

2 tablespoons snipped fresh dill

½ teaspoon whole grain mustard

½ teaspoon freshly ground black pepper

⅛ teaspoon salt

Leaf lettuce, for serving

2 large tomatoes, cut into wedges

8 crispbreads, for serving (we used Wasa)

1. Coarsely chop the eggs and egg whites and place in a medium bowl. Add the celery, cucumber, radishes, scallions, mayonnaise, dill, mustard, pepper, and salt and mix well.
2. Arrange the lettuce leaves on a platter or plates. Mound the salad on top and surround with the tomato wedges. Serve with the crispbreads.

SPRING SALAD WITH PEAS AND MINT

MAKES 8 SERVINGS

- 1 tablespoon sherry or wine vinegar
- 1 tablespoon chopped fresh mint
- 1/4 teaspoon salt
- 1/4 cup + 1 tablespoon olive oil
- 8 cups mixed spring greens
- 1 pound fresh peas, shelled (about 1 cup), or 1/4 pound snow peas, cut up, or a combination
- 5 radishes, sliced
- 1 tablespoon chopped fresh mint

1. In a large bowl, whisk together the vinegar, mint, and salt. Slowly pour in the oil while whisking.
2. Add the greens, peas, radishes, and mint to the dressing, toss, and serve.

PER SERVING:
99 CAL

2 g protein

4 g carbohydrates

9 g fat

1 g saturated fat

2 g fiber

89 mg sodium

HERBED SALAD WITH WALNUTS

PER SERVING:
240 CAL

2 g protein

3 g
carbohydrates

25 g fat

3.5 g
saturated fat

2 g fiber

456 mg sodium

MAKES 4 SERVINGS

6 tablespoons olive oil

2 tablespoons white wine vinegar

3/4 teaspoon salt

8 cups salad greens

1/2 cup chopped fresh herbs (chives, basil, and/or parsley)

1/4 cup roughly chopped walnuts

1. In a large bowl, whisk together the oil, vinegar, and salt.
2. Add the greens and herbs and toss to coat.
3. Top each serving with walnuts.

MIXED GREENS WITH YELLOW PEPPERS

PER SERVING:
109 CAL

2 g protein

5 g
carbohydrates

10 g fat

1.5 g
saturated fat

2 g fiber

117 mg sodium

MAKES 6 SERVINGS

1 yellow bell pepper, thinly sliced

1/2 small red onion, thinly sliced

1/4 cup extra virgin olive oil

2 tablespoons balsamic vinegar

1 clove garlic, crushed or put through garlic press

1/4 teaspoon salt

8 cups salad greens (such as arugula and romaine)

1. In a large salad bowl, combine the bell pepper, onion, oil, vinegar, garlic, and salt. Let stand for 10 minutes.
2. Add the salad greens and toss well.

FENNEL SALAD WITH ORANGE VINAIGRETTE

MAKES 4 SERVINGS

- 2 tablespoons white or red wine vinegar
- 4 teaspoons canola oil
- 1 tablespoon fresh orange juice
- ½ teaspoon Dijon mustard
- ½ bulb fennel
- 1 small red onion
- ½ bag (3 ounces) baby spinach
- 2 cups mixed greens

PER SERVING:

72 CAL

2 g protein

7 g
carbohydrates

5 g fat

0.5 g
saturated fat

3 g fiber

72 mg sodium

1. In a large bowl, whisk together the vinegar, oil, orange juice, and mustard.
2. In a food processor, slice the fennel and onion with the slicing blade, or use a mandoline. (If you'd prefer, use a knife and cut into very thin slices.) Add to the vinaigrette and toss to coat well.
3. Divide the spinach and mixed greens among 4 plates. Top with the fennel mixture.

CHEESE-FREE BEEF ONION SOUP

PER SERVING:
314 CAL

18 g protein

20 g
carbohydrates

18 g fat

2 g
saturated fat

2 g fiber

528 mg sodium

MAKES 4 SERVINGS

4 tablespoons safflower oil

8 ounces beef tenderloin, trimmed

3 large onions, thinly sliced

2 teaspoons sugar

2 cloves garlic, minced

2 tablespoons balsamic vinegar

4 cups fat-free, reduced-sodium beef broth

1 teaspoon Worcestershire sauce

1 slice day-old whole wheat bread

Chives (optional)

1. In a large pot, heat 1 tablespoon of the oil over medium-high heat. Add the beef and cook for about 2 to 3 minutes per side for medium-rare. Transfer to a cutting board and let stand for 5 minutes. Slice across the grain into thin strips. Set aside.

2. Add the remaining 3 tablespoons oil to the pot and reduce the heat to medium. Add the onions and sugar and cook, stirring occasionally, for about 25 minutes, or until golden.

3. Add the garlic and cook for 2 minutes.

4. Increase the heat to medium-high, pour in the vinegar, and bring to a boil. Cook, stirring constantly, for about 1 minute, or until the vinegar is almost completely evaporated.

5. Add the broth and Worcestershire sauce. Bring to a boil, reduce to a simmer, and cook, covered, for 15 minutes.

6. Tear the bread into chunks and whirl in a food processor to form crumbs. Stir the crumbs into the soup and cook for 2 to 3 minutes, or until slightly thickened.

7. Top each serving with an equal portion of the reserved beef slices and garnish with chives (if using).

ITALIAN GREENS AND BEAN SOUP

MAKES 8 SERVINGS

- 1 tablespoon olive oil
- 1 large onion, chopped
- 4 carrots, chopped
- 1 can (14.5 ounces) diced tomatoes with roasted garlic (with juice)
- 2 cans (14.5 ounces each) fat-free, reduced-sodium chicken broth (we used Kitchen Basics)
- 3 cans (15 ounces each) no-salt-added cannellini beans, rinsed and drained
- 1 tablespoon chopped dried rosemary
- 3 cups water
- $\frac{1}{2}$ pound escarole, coarsely chopped
- $\frac{1}{2}$ teaspoon salt
- $\frac{1}{2}$ cup grated Romano cheese
- $\frac{1}{2}$ cup pesto

1. In a large pot, heat the oil over medium-high heat. Cook the onion and carrots, stirring occasionally, for 10 minutes, or until vegetables soften.
2. Add the tomatoes (with juice), the broth, beans, rosemary, and water. Cover and cook about 10 minutes, or until the mixture begins to simmer.
3. Reduce the heat and add the escarole and salt. Cook, uncovered, 15 minutes longer, or until the flavors blend. Stir in the cheese.
4. Spoon 1 tablespoon of the pesto into the center of each serving.

ASPARAGUS SOUP

MAKES 4 SERVINGS

- 2 tablespoons butter
- 8 ounces shiitake (stems removed) or regular mushrooms, sliced
- 1 large onion, chopped
- 2 pounds asparagus, trimmed, roasted or grilled, and cut into pieces ($\frac{1}{2}$ the tips reserved)
- $2\frac{1}{2}$ cups fat-free, reduced-sodium chicken broth
- $\frac{1}{2}$ teaspoon salt
- $\frac{1}{4}$ teaspoon freshly ground black pepper

1. In a medium saucepan, melt 1 tablespoon of the butter over medium-high heat. Cook the mushrooms, stirring occasionally, until golden brown, about 6 minutes. Remove from the pan.
2. In the same saucepan, heat the remaining 1 tablespoon butter. Cook the onion, stirring occasionally, until brown and caramelized, about 12 minutes.
3. In a food processor, combine the onion, asparagus (except the reserved tips), broth, and salt. Process until smooth.
4. Transfer the soup mixture to a pot and add the mushrooms. Bring to a boil. Season with additional salt and the pepper.
5. Garnish with the reserved asparagus tips.

FOUR WAYS TO COOK ASPARAGUS

We recommend roasting or grilling the asparagus to develop its hidden sweet and nutty side. But you can also microwave or steam it.

Grill for a smoky taste. Toss asparagus in a bowl with oil, salt, and pepper. Cook on grill, turning once with tongs, until brown in spots, about 5 minutes.

Microwave for an instant side dish. Cook asparagus spears on high in a microwaveable dish covered with plastic wrap until just tender, 5 to 10 minutes.

Roast it for a sweet, caramelized flavor. Toss asparagus with oil, salt, and pepper on a baking sheet. Put in 450°F oven until browned, about 15 minutes.

Steam it for low calories. Bring $\frac{1}{2}$" of salted water to a boil in a large pan. Simmer the asparagus in a single layer, covered, until tender, about 5 minutes.

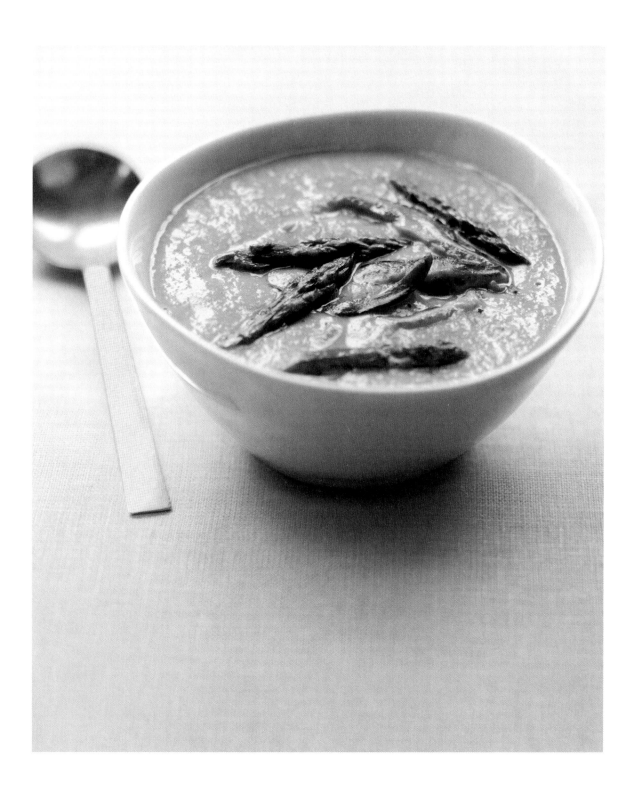

TOMATO-AVOCADO SOUP

PER SERVING:
155 CAL

6 g protein	
19 g carbohydrates	
6 g fat	
1 g saturated fat	
5 g fiber	
500 mg sodium	

MAKES 4 SERVINGS

- 1 can (28 ounces) whole tomatoes
- ½ sweet onion, sliced
- 1 cup reduced-sodium vegetable broth
- 1 cup water
- ½ teaspoon freshly ground black pepper
- 1 cup buttermilk
- ¼ cup fat-free Greek yogurt
- 1 Hass avocado, sliced

1. Preheat the oven to 350°F.
2. Into an 11″ × 17″ baking dish, pour the tomatoes (with juice). Scatter the onion on top and bake for 1 hour, or until the mixture is thick and the onion begins to brown.
3. Transfer the mixture to a blender. Add the broth, water, and pepper and puree until smooth.
4. Heat the soup mixture in a pot over medium-low heat for 5 minutes, or until heated through. Add the buttermilk and stir to combine.
5. Garnish each serving with 1 tablespoon of the yogurt and one-quarter of the avocado slices.

AFRICAN PEANUT SOUP

MAKES 4 SERVINGS

1 tablespoon canola oil

1 onion, chopped

2 ribs celery, chopped

2 carrots, chopped

1 clove garlic, minced

1 tablespoon grated fresh ginger

3 cups reduced-sodium vegetable broth

½ cup creamy natural reduced-fat peanut butter

2 tablespoons freshly squeezed lemon juice

2 tablespoons chopped unsalted peanuts

2 tablespoons chopped fresh cilantro

PER SERVING:

304 CAL

9 g protein

18 g
carbohydrates

22 g fat

3 g
saturated fat

4 g fiber

144 mg sodium

1. In a large pot or Dutch oven, heat the oil over medium-high heat. Cook the onion, celery, and carrots, stirring occasionally, for 5 minutes, or until the onion softens.
2. Add the garlic, ginger, and 2 cups of the broth. Reduce the heat to low, cover, and simmer for 30 minutes, or until the vegetables are very tender.
3. Transfer the soup to a blender or a food processor fitted with a metal blade (in batches, if necessary). Process until smooth.
4. Return the soup to the pot and stir in the peanut butter, lemon juice, and remaining 1 cup broth. Cook for 5 minutes, or until the peanut butter melts and the flavors blend.
5. Garnish each serving with the chopped nuts and cilantro.

SCALLOP AND BROCCOLI CHOWDER

PER SERVING:

230 CAL

23 g protein
23 g carbohydrates
5 g fat
0.5 g saturated fat
4 g fiber
241 mg sodium

MAKES 4 SERVINGS

1 can (15.5 ounces) no-salt-added cannellini beans, rinsed and drained

3 large cloves garlic, slivered

1 tablespoon canola oil

¾ cup water

2 cups fat-free milk

1 teaspoon dried thyme

2 cups broccoli florets, chopped

12 ounces bay scallops

1 small red onion, finely chopped (½ cup), 2 tablespoons reserved for garnish
Ground white pepper

1. In a large nonstick saucepan, combine the beans, garlic, and oil. Cook over medium heat for 3 minutes, or until sizzling and fragrant. Add the water. Cover and simmer for 5 minutes, or until the garlic is tender when pierced with a knife.

2. Transfer the mixture to a blender or a food processor fitted with a metal blade. Process for 2 minutes, scraping the sides of the bowl as needed, until smooth. With the machine running, add about half of the milk through the feed tube, processing just until mixed. Return the mixture to the saucepan.

3. Add the remaining milk and the thyme. Stir to combine. Bring to a simmer. Add the broccoli and continue to simmer for 3 minutes. Add the scallops and all but 2 tablespoons of the onion. Simmer for 3 to 4 minutes, or until the scallops are opaque. Ladle into bowls. Garnish with the reserved onion and season with the pepper.

ITALIAN CHICKEN-ARTICHOKE-RICE SOUP

MAKES 4 SERVINGS

- 1 tablespoon canola oil
- 1 medium onion, chopped (about 1 cup)
- 1 teaspoon dried oregano
- 4 cups fat-free, reduced-sodium vegetable or chicken broth
- 2 cups water
- 1 can (14 ounces) no-salt-added diced tomatoes, with juice
- 6 tablespoons instant brown rice
- $\frac{1}{4}$ teaspoon salt
- 8 ounces cooked boneless, skinless chicken breast, chopped (1$\frac{1}{2}$ cups)
- 1 package (9 ounces) frozen artichoke hearts, thawed and chopped
- $\frac{1}{4}$ cup chopped Italian parsley
  Freshly ground black pepper
- 4 teaspoons grated Parmesan cheese

PER SERVING:
250 CAL
22 g protein

22 g
carbohydrates

7 g fat

1 g
saturated fat

6 g fiber

415 mg sodium

1. Heat a large pot over medium heat. Add the oil and heat for 1 minute. Add the onion and oregano. Stir and cover. Cook, stirring occasionally, for 3 minutes, or until the onion starts to soften.
2. Stir in the broth, water, tomatoes (with juice), rice, and salt. Bring almost to a boil and then reduce the heat. Simmer for 10 minutes, stirring occasionally, until the rice is tender.
3. Add the chicken and artichokes. Simmer for 3 minutes, just until heated through. Stir in the parsley and season to taste with pepper. Ladle into 4 bowls and sprinkle 1 teaspoon of the cheese over each.

TURKEY, SWEET POTATO, AND CRANBERRY STEW

PER SERVING:
412 CAL

53 g protein

35 g carbohydrates

6 g fat

2 g saturated fat

4 g fiber

909 mg sodium

MAKES 4 SERVINGS

- 3 pounds turkey drumsticks, skin removed
- 1 small onion, chopped
- 1 tablespoon honey
- 1 tablespoon cider vinegar
- 1½ teaspoons finely chopped fresh ginger
- 1 teaspoon salt
- ½ teaspoon freshly ground black pepper
- 1 cup fat-free, reduced sodium chicken broth (we used Kitchen Basics)
- 1 pound sweet potatoes, peeled and cut into 1" chunks
- ½ cup dried cranberries
- 2 tablespoons all-purpose flour

1. In a large slow cooker, combine the turkey, onion, honey, vinegar, ginger, salt, pepper, and broth. Cover and cook on low for 5 hours. Add the potatoes and cranberries. Cook until the potatoes are tender, for 45 minutes more.
2. Remove the turkey and pull the meat from the bones. Pour one-quarter of the liquid into a small pot and whisk in the flour until smooth. Slowly whisk in the remaining liquid.
3. Toss the meat, potatoes, and cranberries with the gravy and reheat if necessary.

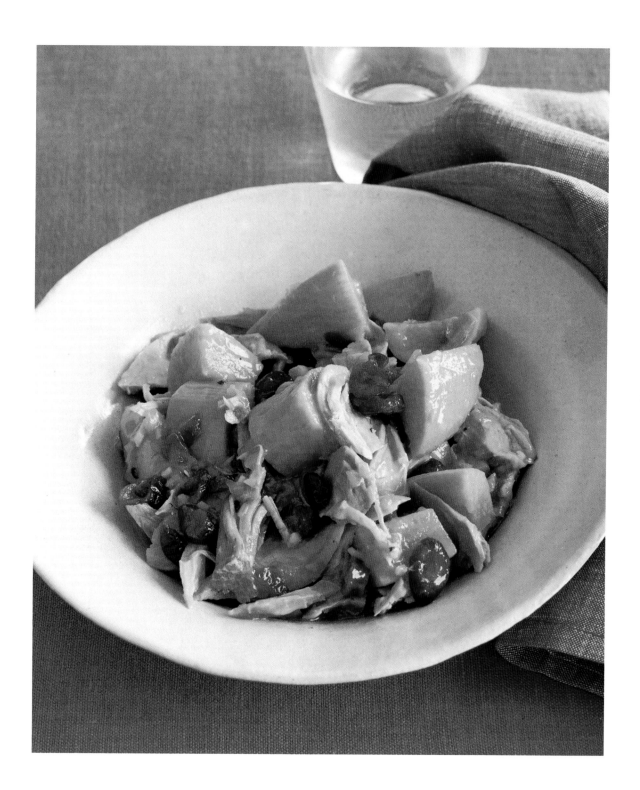

SIDE DISHES

GREEN BEANS WITH TOMATOES AND BASIL

MAKES 6 SERVINGS

1 pound green beans, cut into 2" pieces
2 tablespoons olive oil
3 cloves garlic, sliced
1 cup red and/or yellow cherry tomatoes, halved
2 tablespoons balsamic vinegar
1 tablespoon chopped fresh basil or 1 teaspoon dried basil
½ teaspoon salt

1. Fill a large skillet with ¾" water and bring to a boil. Add the beans and cook for 6 minutes or until just tender. Drain and set aside. Wipe the skillet dry.
2. Heat the oil in the same skillet over medium-high heat. Cook the garlic for 2 minutes. Add the tomatoes and cook for 3 minutes, or until browned. Stir in the vinegar, cooking for 1 minute to loosen the brown bits. Stir in the beans, basil, and salt. Cook for 1 minute, or until heated through.

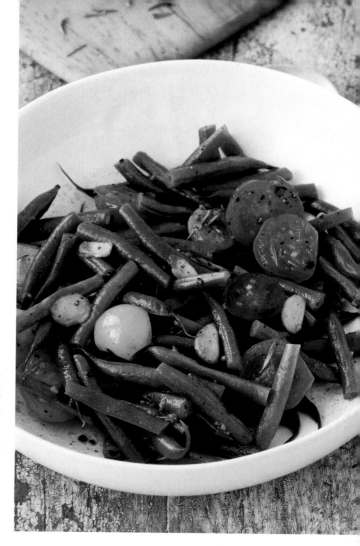

PER SERVING:
73 CAL

2 g protein

7 g carbohydrates

5 g fat

1 g saturated fat

2 g fiber

201 mg sodium

CORN AND ZUCCHINI WITH HERBED OIL

PER SERVING:

235 CAL

5 g protein
23 g carbohydrates
16 g fat
2.5 g saturated fat
3 g fiber
26 mg sodium

MAKES 4 SERVINGS

- ¼ cup extra virgin olive oil
- 2 tablespoons finely chopped fresh chives
- 2 tablespoons finely chopped parsley
- 4 ears corn, husked
- 4 small zucchini, halved lengthwise, then crosswise
  Salt
  Freshly ground black pepper

1. Coat a grill rack with cooking spray. Preheat the grill to medium.
2. In a small bowl, combine the oil, chives, and parsley. Brush the corn and zucchini very lightly with the oil mixture and season with salt and black pepper.
3. Grill the corn for 2 minutes. Add the zucchini to the grill and continue cooking until both are tender, about 10 minutes longer, turning occasionally. Drizzle any remaining oil over all before serving.

BALSAMIC ROASTED CARROTS

MAKES 2 SERVINGS

  8 medium carrots, quartered lengthwise

  2 tablespoons extra virgin olive oil

  1 tablespoon balsamic vinegar

  ½ teaspoon salt

  ¼ teaspoon freshly ground black pepper

1. Preheat the oven to 450°F.
2. In a roasting pan, combine the carrots, 1 tablespoon of the oil, the vinegar, salt, and pepper. Toss to coat. Roast for 20 to 25 minutes, tossing occasionally, until lightly caramelized and tender but still firm. Drizzle with the remaining tablespoon of oil.

PER SERVING:

232 CAL

2 g protein

25 g
carbohydrates

15 g fat

2 g
saturated fat

7 g fiber

650 mg sodium

MUSHROOM RAGOUT

PER SERVING:

129 CAL

8 g protein	
12 g carbohydrates	
6 g fat	
2 g saturated fat	
2 g fiber	
161 mg sodium	

MAKES 4 SERVINGS

- 2 teaspoons canola oil
- 1 small onion, finely chopped
- 1¼ pounds baby bella mushrooms, sliced
- ½ teaspoon finely chopped fresh rosemary
- ⅛ teaspoon salt
- 2 tablespoons white whole wheat flour
- 2 tablespoons nonfat dry milk
- 1 tablespoon ground flaxseed
- ⅛ teaspoon grated fresh nutmeg
- 1 cup buttermilk
- ¼ cup grated Parmesan cheese
- 1⅓ cups shredded reduced-fat Swiss cheese

1. Heat a nonstick skillet over medium-high heat. Add the oil and heat for 1 minute. Add the onion. Cook, stirring occasionally, for 2 minutes, or until the onion starts to soften. Add the mushrooms, rosemary, and salt. Stir. Cover and cook for 4 minutes, or until the mushrooms give up liquid. Remove the cover and cook for 4 minutes, or until the liquid becomes syrupy.

2. Meanwhile, in a bowl, combine the flour, dry milk, flaxseed, and nutmeg. Gradually add the buttermilk, whisking constantly, until smooth. Add to the skillet, stirring constantly, for 3 minutes, or until thickened. Remove from the heat. Stir in the cheeses until the Swiss melts.

SAFFRON RICE WITH PISTACHIOS

MAKES 4 SERVINGS

- ½ teaspoon saffron threads
- 1 tablespoon + 2¼ cups water
- ½ cup pistachios
- 1 teaspoon olive oil
- ½ teaspoon salt
- 1½ cups instant brown rice

PER SERVING:

229 CAL

6 g protein

30 g
carbohydrates

10 g fat

1 g
saturated fat

3 g fiber

300 mg sodium

1. In a small bowl, soak the saffron in 1 tablespoon of water for 20 minutes. Use the back of a spoon to mash the threads.

2. In a large nonstick skillet, toast the pistachios over medium heat, stirring often, for 3 to 4 minutes, or until lightly browned and fragrant. Tip onto a plate and let cool.

3. In a saucepan, bring the oil, salt, and remaining 2¼ cups of water to a boil over medium-high heat. Reduce the heat to low, add the rice and the saffron mixture, and cook, covered, for 5 minutes. Turn off the heat and let the rice sit for 5 minutes.

4. Fluff the rice with a fork and stir in the pistachios.

ROASTED POTATOES
WITH BLUE CHEESE AND WALNUTS

PER SERVING:

243 CAL

8 g protein
21 g carbohydrates
15 g fat
4 g saturated fat
3 g fiber
280 mg sodium

MAKES 4 SERVINGS

1 pound thin-skinned baby potatoes, halved

1½ teaspoons olive oil

¼ teaspoon freshly ground black pepper

⅛ teaspoon salt

½ cup coarsely chopped walnuts

2 ounces crumbled blue cheese

2 scallions, thinly sliced

1. Preheat the oven to 425°F. Coat a 9″ × 9″ baking dish with cooking spray or line with parchment paper.

2. Place the potatoes in the prepared dish and toss with the oil, pepper, and salt. Turn the potatoes cut side down in the pan. Roast for 30 to 35 minutes, or until very tender and lightly golden on the underside.

3. Meanwhile, in a small baking pan or ovenproof skillet, place the walnuts and transfer to the oven to toast for 6 to 8 minutes. Tip into a bowl and let cool. Add the blue cheese and scallions and crumble with your fingers.

4. When the potatoes are done, turn them over and sprinkle them evenly with the walnut mixture. Bake for 5 minutes longer, or until the cheese is melted.

PROSCIUTTO-GRILLED ASPARAGUS

MAKES 6 SERVINGS

24 large asparagus spears, trimmed

2 tablespoons olive oil

Salt

Freshly ground black pepper

12 large, paper-thin slices prosciutto

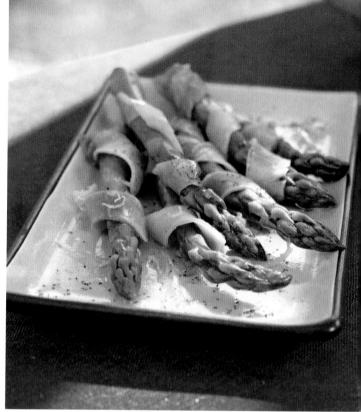

1. Coat a ridged grill pan or barbecue grill with olive oil spray and heat to medium. Place the asparagus on a plate; drizzle with the oil and season to taste with salt and pepper. Roll in the oil to evenly coat.

2. Grill the asparagus, turning once or twice, for about 5 minutes, or until lightly charred and just tender. Transfer to a plate and let cool.

3. Cut each slice of prosciutto in half. Roll a half slice of prosciutto around each asparagus spear.

PER SERVING:

113 CAL

9 g protein

4 g carbohydrates

8 g fat

2 g saturated fat

1 g fiber

751 mg sodium

LIGHT AND LUSCIOUS EGGPLANT PARM

PER SERVING:

300 CAL

| 10 g protein |
| 24 g carbohydrates |
| 11 g fiber |
| 21 g fat |
| 5 g saturated fat |
| 11 g fiber |
| 827 mg sodium |

MAKES 4 SERVINGS

2-3 small eggplants (about 2¼ pounds), cut into ¼"-thick slices

¼ cup + 1½ teaspoons olive oil

1 teaspoon salt + more for seasoning

1 clove garlic, thinly sliced

2 pounds plum tomatoes or 1 can (28 ounces) tomatoes, chopped

20 fresh basil leaves

½ teaspoon freshly ground black pepper + more for seasoning

¾ cup freshly grated Parmesan cheese

1. Preheat the oven to 400°F. Generously oil 2 nonstick baking sheets.
2. Put the eggplant on the prepared baking sheets and brush the tops with ¼ cup of the oil. Sprinkle with ¼ teaspoon of the salt. Bake for 30 minutes, or until softened.
3. In a medium saucepan, heat the remaining 1½ teaspoons of oil over medium-high heat. Add the garlic and cook, stirring frequently, for 1 minute.
4. Add the tomatoes, basil, pepper, and remaining ¾ teaspoon of salt and cook until the sauce is thickened and reduced to about 2 cups, for about 15 minutes. Season with the salt and pepper.
5. Transfer the tomato mixture to the food processor and puree until nearly smooth.
6. Coat the bottom of an 8" × 8" baking pan with ½ cup of the sauce. Add one-third of the eggplant, and top with another ½ cup of the sauce and 3 tablespoons of the cheese. Repeat twice (eggplant, sauce, cheese), ending with remaining 6 tablespoons cheese.
7. Bake until browned, for about 30 minutes. Let rest for 10 minutes before serving.

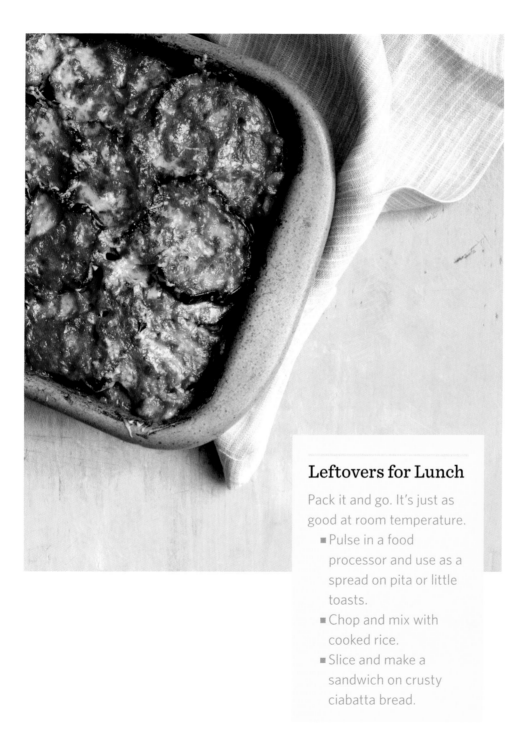

Leftovers for Lunch

Pack it and go. It's just as good at room temperature.

- Pulse in a food processor and use as a spread on pita or little toasts.
- Chop and mix with cooked rice.
- Slice and make a sandwich on crusty ciabatta bread.

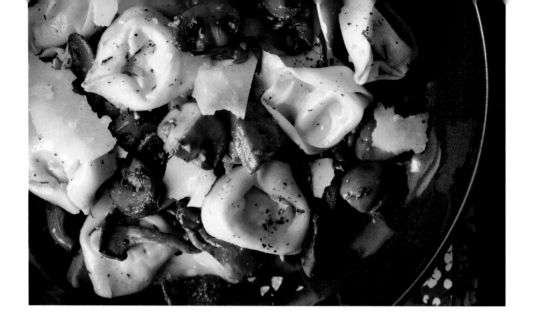

TORTELLINI WITH MUSHROOMS

PER SERVING:

306 CAL

9 g protein

31 g
carbohydrates

15 g fat

3 g
saturated fat

2 g fiber

493 mg sodium

MAKES 4 SERVINGS

  2 tablespoons olive oil

½ pound mixed mushrooms, halved (we used regular white mushrooms and stemmed shiitakes)

  4 teaspoons minced fresh garlic

¾ teaspoon dried thyme

½ teaspoon salt

¼ teaspoon freshly ground black pepper

½ cup Madeira or dry sherry

  8 ounces fresh cheese tortellini

  1 tablespoon extra virgin olive oil

    Grated or shaved Parmesan cheese (optional)

1. In a large nonstick skillet, heat the olive oil. Cook the mushrooms, stirring frequently, until golden, for about 8 minutes. Add the garlic and thyme and cook for 1 minute. Season with the salt and pepper. Add the Madeira or dry sherry, reduce the heat, and simmer for 5 minutes.
2. Cook the tortellini according to the package directions. Add the pasta to the warm mushrooms and simmer for 2 minutes. Stir in 1 tablespoon extra virgin olive oil and sprinkle with the cheese (if using).

LINGUINE WITH WALNUT-TOMATO PESTO

MAKES 4 SERVINGS

1 cup fresh basil leaves

¼ cup walnut pieces

2 cloves garlic

6 oil-packed sun-dried tomatoes

2 tablespoons grated Parmesan cheese

½ teaspoon salt

¼ teaspoon red-pepper flakes

6 tablespoons olive oil

12 ounces linguine

PER SERVING:
460 CAL

10 g protein

45 g carbohydrates

27 g fat

4 g saturated fat

3 g fiber

345 mg sodium

1. In the food processor, chop the basil, walnuts, and garlic. Add the tomatoes, cheese, salt, and red-pepper flakes. Pulse to combine, scraping down sides. Drizzle in the oil with the machine running. Process to a coarse paste.
2. Cook the pasta according to the package directions. Add 1 cup of the cooking water to the food processor and pulse until smooth.
3. Drain the pasta and return to the warm pot. Toss the pesto with the pasta.

GIANT MUSHROOMS STUFFED WITH GREENS AND MOZZARELLA

PER SERVING:
331 CAL

18 g protein

20 g
carbohydrates

22 g fat

5.5 g
saturated fat

5 g fiber

794 mg sodium

MAKES 4 SERVINGS

- 2 tablespoons canola oil
- 1 pound Swiss chard, trimmed, stems removed and sliced crosswise, and leaves chopped
- 2 cloves garlic, crushed
- ½ teaspoon salt
- 1 bunch scallions (about 6), bulbs and greens separated and sliced
- 8 portobello mushroom caps (1⅔ pounds total)
- ½ cup drained canned fire-roasted diced tomatoes
- 5 ounces part-skim mozzarella or smoked mozzarella, coarsely grated
- 2 tablespoons finely chopped fresh parsley
  Freshly ground black pepper
- ½ cup crushed unsalted roasted cashews

1. Preheat the oven to 400°F.
2. In a large frying pan, heat 1½ teaspoons of the oil over medium-high heat. Cook the chard stems, garlic, and salt for 5 minutes. Stir in the scallion bulbs and chard leaves. Cook until tender, about 12 minutes, stirring occasionally. Remove from the heat.
3. In a medium bowl, coat the mushrooms with the remaining 4½ teaspoons oil and lightly sprinkle all over with salt. Put on a large baking sheet.
4. Stir the tomatoes, scallion greens, cheese, and parsley into the chard mixture and season with pepper to taste. Fill the mushrooms with the chard stuffing. Bake until hot, for 15 to 20 minutes. Sprinkle with the cashews before serving.

SUPERFOOD: MUSHROOMS

Mushrooms contain cancer-fighting selenium. Just two provide 56 percent of the daily recommendation. Portobellos are the perfect stuffing mushroom. They're just regular brown mushrooms, all grown up.

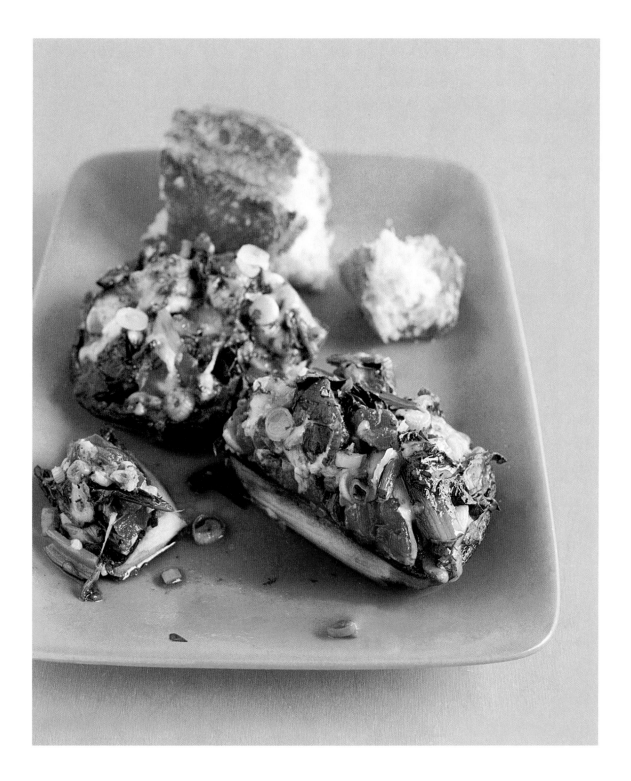

EVERYDAY SOUFFLÉ

PER SERVING:

251 CAL

22 g protein	
23 g carbohydrates	
7 g fat	
4 g saturated fat	
5 g fiber	
452 mg sodium	

MAKES 4 SERVINGS

- 1 tablespoon dried bread crumbs
- 1 pound broccoli, cut into florets
- 3 eggs, separated
- 1½ cups fat-free milk
- ⅓ cup all-purpose flour
- ¾ teaspoon dry mustard
- 1 clove garlic, minced
- ½ cup grated Romano cheese
- 3 egg whites
- ⅛ teaspoon cream of tartar

1. Preheat the oven to 375°F. Coat a 2-quart soufflé dish with cooking spray. Add the bread crumbs and shake to coat.
2. Place a steamer basket in a large pot with 2″ of water. Bring to a boil over high heat. Place the broccoli in the basket and steam for 8 minutes, or until very tender. Drain and rinse under cold water. Place on a clean kitchen towel to dry. Finely chop the broccoli and place in a large bowl.
3. In a small bowl, whisk together the 3 egg yolks and set aside.
4. In a medium saucepan, whisk together the milk, flour, mustard, and garlic. Bring to a boil over medium heat. Reduce the heat and simmer, stirring constantly, for 3 minutes, or until slightly thickened. Remove from the heat. Whisk some of the milk mixture into the egg yolks. Whisk the egg yolk mixture into the saucepan. Cook for 2 minutes, or until thick. Pour into the bowl with the broccoli and stir in the cheese.
5. In a large mixing bowl, beat all 6 egg whites and the cream of tartar with an electric mixer on high speed until stiff, glossy peaks form, occasionally scraping down the sides of the bowl with a rubber spatula.
6. Stir about one-third of the whites into the broccoli mixture. Fold in the remaining whites. Pour into the prepared dish. Bake for 30 to 40 minutes, or until puffed and golden.

SPINACH, TOMATO, AND SWISS CHEESE QUICHE

MAKES 4 SERVINGS

PER SERVING:
169 CAL

15 g protein

16 g
carbohydrates

5 g fat

1 g
saturated fat

4 g fiber

560 mg sodium

- 1 tablespoon water
- 8 cups fresh baby spinach
- 4 scallions, thinly sliced
- 2 egg whites
- 2 tablespoons ground flaxseed
- 2 slices (¾ ounce each) reduced-fat Swiss cheese, cut into slivers
- 2 tablespoons grated Parmesan cheese
- ½ cup canned diced tomatoes, drained and patted dry
- 2 eggs
- 1½ cups fat-free milk
- 2 tablespoons nonfat dry milk
- Pinch of ground fresh nutmeg
- ¼ teaspoon salt
- ¼ teaspoon freshly ground black pepper

1. Preheat the oven to 350°F. Coat a 9" quiche or pie dish with cooking spray.
2. Heat the water in a nonstick skillet. Add the spinach and scallions. Toss. Cover and cook for 2 minutes, or until wilted. Drain. Allow to cool. Squeeze very dry. Transfer to a work surface and very finely chop the mixture.
3. In a bowl, beat 1 of the egg whites. Add the flaxseed and spinach mixture. Stir to combine. Transfer to the prepared dish. Press with the back of a fork to cover the bottom and sides of the pan. Top with the cheeses. Scatter on the tomatoes.
4. In the same bowl, beat the 2 eggs and the remaining egg white. Add the milk, dry milk, nutmeg, salt, and pepper. Beat to combine. Pour carefully into the pan.
5. Bake for 30 minutes, or until golden and set. Allow to sit for 10 minutes before serving.

MOCK ITALIAN MEATBALLS

PER SERVING:

244 CAL

12 g protein

23 g carbohydrates

12 g fat

4 g saturated fat

10 g fiber

645 mg sodium

MAKES 4 SERVINGS

- 1 can (14.5 ounces) diced tomatoes
- 2 teaspoons dried oregano

  Freshly ground black pepper
- 2½ pounds globe or Japanese eggplant, peeled and cut into ½"-thick slices
- 2 cloves garlic
- ½ cup grated Pecorino cheese
- ¼ cup finely chopped parsley
- ¼ cup ground flaxseed
- ¼ cup nonfat dry milk
- ¼ teaspoon salt
- 1 tablespoon olive oil

1. Preheat the oven to 375°F. Coat a 13" × 9" baking dish with cooking spray.
2. Add the tomatoes to the prepared baking dish. Sprinkle with the oregano and sprinkle generously with the pepper. Set aside.
3. On a large microwaveable plate or directly on a glass turntable, place the eggplant in a single layer. Microwave for 10 minutes, turning once, or until very soft. (This might have to be done in 2 batches.) Allow to cool to room temperature. Rinse with cold water. Drain and squeeze the eggplant dry.
4. In a blender or food processor, pulse the garlic until finely chopped. Add the eggplant, Pecorino, parsley, flaxseed, dry milk, and salt. Pulse, scraping the sides of the bowl as needed, until ground. Shape the mixture into 8 balls. Set in the prepared pan. Drizzle evenly with the oil.
5. Bake for about 25 minutes, or until the balls are heated through and the sauce is bubbling.

KANSAS CITY–STYLE BARBECUED TOFU
WITH COLLARD GREENS

MAKES 4 SERVINGS

- 1 teaspoon canola oil
- 1 small onion, finely chopped
- 1 block tofu (14 ounces), drained, cut into 8 cutlets, frozen, thawed, and squeezed dry
- ¾ cup no-salt-added tomato sauce
- 3 tablespoons molasses
- ½ teaspoon hot-pepper sauce
- ¼ teaspoon dry mustard
- ⅛ teaspoon ground cloves
- 6 cups coarsely chopped fresh collard greens

PER SERVING:
243 CAL

18 g protein	
24 g carbohydrates	
10 g fat	
1 g saturated fat	
5 g fiber	
54 mg sodium	

1. Heat a large nonstick skillet over medium heat. Add the oil and onion. Cook, stirring occasionally, for 2 minutes, or until the onion starts to soften. Scrape the onion to the side. Add the tofu. Fry for 2 to 3 minutes, or until golden on the bottom. Flip and fry for 2 minutes more.

2. In a small bowl, stir together the tomato sauce, molasses, hot-pepper sauce, dry mustard, and cloves. Stir into the skillet. Scatter the collards on top. Cover and simmer for 5 minutes.

3. Stir the mixture gently. Cover and continue to simmer for 10 minutes, or until the collards are very tender. Serve additional hot-pepper sauce at the table.

CHICKEN AND TURKEY MAIN DISHES

CHICKEN WITH GRAPEFRUIT

MAKES 4 SERVINGS

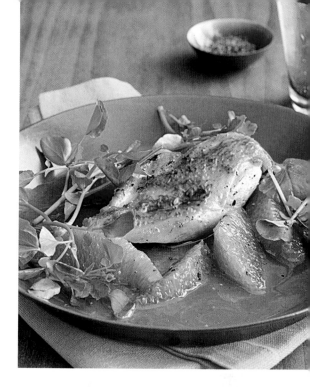

- 4 boneless chicken breasts
- ½ teaspoon dried thyme
- ½ teaspoon salt
- ¼ teaspoon freshly ground black pepper
- 2 tablespoons olive oil
- ¼ cup dry white wine
- ¼ cup fat-free, reduced-sodium chicken broth (we used Kitchen Basics)
- 3 tablespoons grapefruit juice
- 2 teaspoons honey
- 3 cups trimmed fresh watercress
- 2 grapefruit, cut into segments

1. Season the chicken with the thyme and half of the salt and pepper.
2. In a skillet, heat the oil over medium-high heat. Brown the chicken, for 6 minutes a side. Add the wine, broth, grapefruit juice, and honey. Simmer until reduced to ⅓ cup. Season with the remaining salt and pepper.
3. Put the watercress and grapefruit on plates. Top with the chicken and sauce.

PER SERVING:

266 CAL

27 g protein

15 g carbohydrates

10 g fat

2 g saturated fat

2 g fiber

438 mg sodium

INSTANT TERIYAKI CHICKEN

PER SERVING:

201 CAL

29 g protein

8 g
carbohydrates

6 g fat

1.5 g
saturated fat

1 g fiber

657 mg sodium

MAKES 4 SERVINGS

- 2 tablespoons reduced sodium soy sauce
- 1½ tablespoons honey
- 1 tablespoon tomato paste
- 4 bone-in, skinless chicken thighs (about 5 ounces each)
- 1 teaspoon sesame seeds, toasted (optional)

1. Coat a grill rack or broiler pan with cooking spray. Preheat the grill or broiler to high.
2. In a medium bowl, stir together the soy sauce, honey, and tomato paste. Add the chicken and turn to coat all surfaces.
3. Put the chicken on the grill or in an ovenproof pan under the broiler.
4. Cook the chicken until well browned, for about 4 minutes on the grill or 10 minutes under the broiler. Flip and brown the second side until cooked through, for about 2 minutes on the grill or 4 minutes under the broiler. Sprinkle with sesame seeds (if using).

SHOPPING TIP

Buy tomato paste in a tube. It lasts indefinitely in the refrigerator. Or freeze leftovers from a can in tablespoon-size portions on a sheet of wax paper, peel them off, and store frozen in a resealable plastic bag.

INDIAN-STYLE CHICKEN

MAKES 4 SERVINGS

2½ pounds mixed bone-in chicken pieces (thighs, drumsticks, or breasts), skin removed

½ cup plain yogurt

1 tablespoon freshly squeezed lemon juice

1 tablespoon grated fresh ginger

3 cloves garlic, minced

2 teaspoons ground coriander

1½ teaspoons paprika

1 teaspoon ground cumin

1 teaspoon salt

¼ teaspoon ground red pepper

2 tablespoons canola oil

1. With a sharp knife, cut three or four ¼"-deep slashes in each piece of chicken.
2. In a large bowl, combine the yogurt, lemon juice, ginger, garlic, coriander, paprika, cumin, salt, and red pepper. Stir until well combined. Add the chicken to the bowl and turn to coat well with the marinade. Marinate the chicken for 30 minutes at room temperature or refrigerate, covered, up to 24 hours. (If the chicken is refrigerated, remove it about 30 minutes before cooking.)
3. Coat a broiler pan or grill rack with cooking spray. Preheat the broiler or grill.
4. With tongs, pick up one piece of chicken at a time and let any excess marinade drip back into the bowl. Put the chicken on the broiler pan or grill rack and brush the pieces with 1 tablespoon of the oil. Discard the marinade.
5. If broiling, cook the chicken about 6" from the heat source until brown, for about 8 minutes. Remove from the oven. Turn the pieces over and brush with the remaining 1 tablespoon of oil. Broil the chicken until done, about 6 minutes longer for breasts and 8 minutes longer for thighs and drumsticks. If grilling, cook the chicken over medium-high heat for 10 minutes. Turn, baste with the oil, and cook for 10 minutes longer for breasts and 12 minutes longer for thighs and drumsticks.

QUICK CHICKEN DIVAN

PER SERVING:

501 CAL

40 g protein

51 g
carbohydrates

15 g fat

7 g
saturated fat

4 g fiber

773 mg sodium

MAKES 4 SERVINGS

- 8 ounces gemelli, rotini, or ziti
- 1/2 pound broccoli, tops cut into florets and stems peeled and sliced
- 1 tablespoon butter
- 2 teaspoons dried basil
- 4 teaspoons all-purpose flour
- 1 cup fat-free, reduced-sodium chicken broth (we used Kitchen Basics)
- 2/3 cup 2% milk
- 3/4 teaspoon salt
- 1 small rotisserie chicken, meat pulled off the bone (2 1/2–3 cups total)
- 1/2 cup shredded reduced-fat Cheddar cheese

  Salt and freshly ground black pepper

1. Prepare the pasta according to the package directions. Add the broccoli during last 5 minutes of cooking. Drain.
2. Melt the butter with the basil in the pasta pot and stir in the flour. When light brown, whisk in the broth, milk, and salt. Bring to a boil. Toss with the chicken, pasta/broccoli mixture, and cheese. Season with salt and pepper.

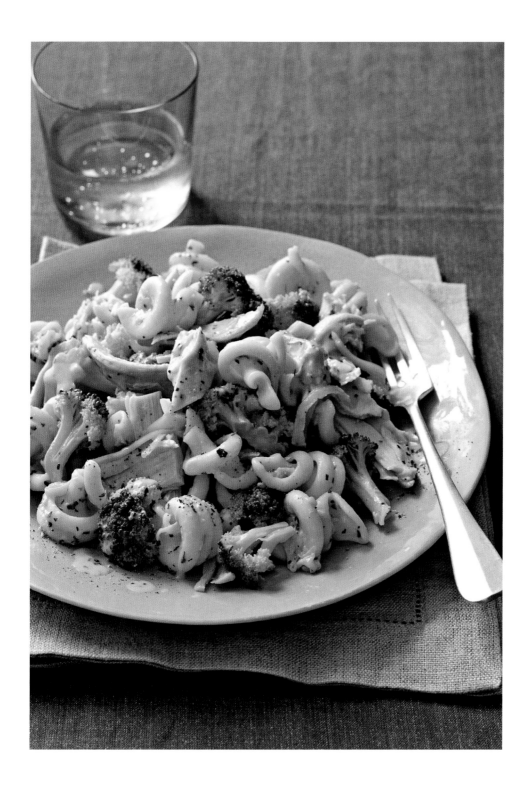

CHICKEN AND SAUSAGE SKEWERS

PER SERVING:

369 CAL

27 g protein

11 g
carbohydrates

24 g fat

7 g
saturated fat

2 g fiber

612 mg sodium

MAKES 4 SERVINGS

10 ounces boneless, skinless chicken breasts, cut into 1½" pieces

6 ounces chorizo, linguica, or hot Italian sausage, cut into 1½" lengths

2 red bell peppers, cut into 1½"-wide strips

1 medium onion, cut into 8 wedges

¼ cup orange juice

½ teaspoon grated orange zest

2 tablespoons finely chopped fresh oregano or 2 teaspoons dried

1 tablespoon smoked or plain paprika

1½ tablespoons extra virgin olive oil

4 cloves garlic, crushed or put through garlic press

1. In a large bowl, combine the chicken, sausage, bell peppers, onion, orange juice, orange zest, oregano, paprika, olive oil, and garlic. Chill for 15 to 30 minutes.
2. Coat a grill rack with cooking spray. Preheat the grill to medium.
3. Thread the chicken and sausage onto skewers. Sprinkle with salt and pepper. Grill until the chicken is just done, for about 10 minutes, turning occasionally.
4. Meanwhile, grill the peppers and onion until tender, for 5 to 6 minutes. Serve the skewers with the peppers and onion.

Grilling Gear

We're fans of the grill basket for keeping small ingredients like cut-up vegetables out of the fire, but many outdoor cooks prefer the ease of a vegetable grill grate, which works, too.

EASIEST EVER BAKED CHICKEN

MAKES 4 SERVINGS

8	chicken drumsticks (about 2 pounds total)
¾	teaspoon salt
¼	teaspoon freshly ground black pepper
¼	teaspoon paprika
⅛	teaspoon ground red pepper (optional)
1	tablespoon olive or canola oil

1. Preheat the oven to 450°F.
2. On a rimmed baking sheet, place the drumsticks close together. Sprinkle with the salt, black pepper, paprika, and red pepper (if using). Drizzle with the oil. Toss the drumsticks to distribute the oil and seasonings evenly. Arrange the drumsticks 1" apart so they'll brown nicely.
3. Bake until browned and cooked through, for about 25 to 30 minutes.

TASTY SWITCH

Go light or dark. You can substitute chicken thighs for the drumsticks, or use four of each. If you prefer white meat, use bone-in split breasts and bake for 30 minutes.

PER SERVING:
275 CAL

29 g protein

0 g carbohydrates

17 g fat

4 g saturated fat

0 g fiber

562 mg sodium

MU SHU CHICKEN

MAKES 4 SERVINGS

- ½ teaspoon cornstarch
- 1 tablespoon reduced-sodium soy sauce
- 2 tablespoons dry sherry
- 2 tablespoons hoisin
- 2 teaspoons canola oil
- 1 tablespoon finely chopped fresh ginger
- 1 tablespoon minced fresh garlic
- 1 bag (14 ounces) coleslaw mix
- ½ cup chopped scallions
- 2 cups shredded rotisserie chicken
- 1 teaspoon toasted sesame oil
- 4 low-carb, whole wheat tortillas (8" diameter)

1. In a small bowl, whisk together the cornstarch, soy sauce, dry sherry, and hoisin.
2. In a large nonstick skillet, heat the canola oil over medium-high heat. Add the ginger and garlic and stir constantly for 1 minute. Add the coleslaw mix and scallions and stir constantly until just wilted, for about 3 minutes. Add the chicken and the soy sauce mixture. Toss until heated through. Drizzle with the sesame oil.
3. Warm the tortillas in the microwave oven. Serve the chicken mixture wrapped in the tortillas, and, if desired, with additional hoisin to spread on the tortillas and chopped scallions to sprinkle over the filling.

QUICK CHICKEN ZITI

MAKES 4 SERVINGS

- 8 ounces ziti (about 3 cups)
- 1 pound chicken breast tenders or thinly sliced boneless, skinless chicken breasts, cut into bite-size chunks
- ¼ teaspoon garlic powder
- 3 small zucchini, trimmed, halved lengthwise, and cut into ¼"-thick slices
- 1 tablespoon olive oil
- 1 cup chunky tomato sauce
- 2 ounces thinly sliced prosciutto, torn into small pieces
- ⅔ cup grated Parmesan cheese

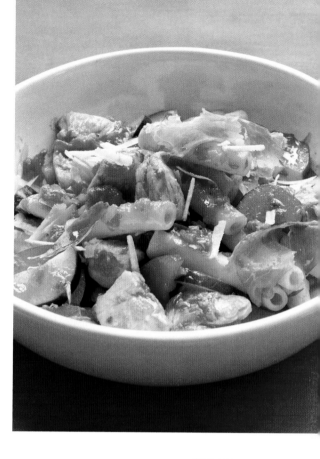

1. Prepare the pasta according to the package directions.
2. Meanwhile, sprinkle the chicken with the garlic powder.
3. Add the zucchini to the pasta cooking water about 1½ minutes before the pasta is done. Drain the pasta and zucchini.
4. In the pasta pot, heat the oil over high heat. Add the chicken and cook, stirring occasionally, for 4 minutes. Pour the tomato sauce over the chicken and simmer until cooked through, for about 3 minutes longer.
5. Add the zucchini and pasta to the chicken and bring just to a simmer, stirring often. Mix in the prosciutto. Top each serving with the cheese.

PER SERVING:
487 CAL

| 42 g protein |
| 49 g carbohydrates |
| 13 g fat |
| 4 g saturated fat |
| 3 g fiber |
| 952 mg sodium |

Cook's Trick

Stretch high-calorie cheese: Grate Parmesan on the coarse side of the grater, and sprinkle the cheese on top rather than stirring it into the pasta. You'll see those big shreds clearly, and the eye can fool the tastebuds and tummy.

CHICKEN REUBEN QUESADILLAS

PER SERVING:

399 CAL

28 g protein
34 g carbohydrates
19 g fat
5.5 g saturated fat
3 g fiber
924 mg sodium

MAKES 4 SERVINGS

- 4 flour tortillas (8" diameter)
- ⅓ cup bottled Russian dressing
- 6 ounces reduced-fat Swiss cheese
- 1 cup drained low-sodium sauerkraut
- 6 ounces sliced reduced-sodium deli chicken breast
- 1 teaspoon canola oil

1. Preheat the oven to 425°F. Brush a baking sheet lightly with canola oil.
2. Place the tortillas on a work surface. Spread the dressing on the tortillas. Divide the cheese, sauerkraut, and chicken and cover half of each tortilla. Fold the other half over the filling and put on the prepared baking sheet. Brush the tops and edges with 1 teaspoon of canola oil and bake for 10 minutes. Flip the quesadillas, transfer to a cutting board, and let rest for 5 minutes. Cut each into 3 wedges.

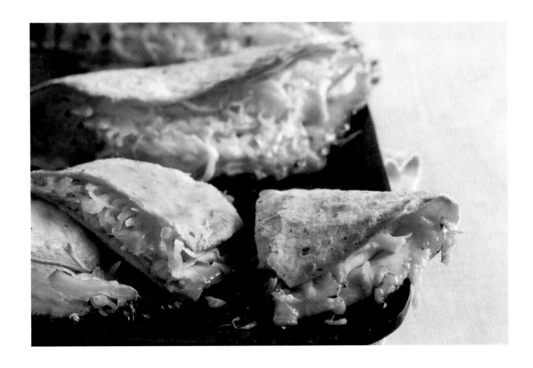

GRILLED TURKEY AND CRANBERRY SANDWICH

MAKES 4 SERVINGS

- 4 teaspoons olive oil
- 8 slices whole grain bread
- 4 ounces pepper jack or mozzarella cheese, sliced
- 8 ounces roast turkey, sliced
- ⅓ cup leftover cranberry sauce, strained if runny

PER SERVING:

432 CAL

30 g protein

41 g carbohydrates

16 g fat

6.5 g saturated fat

5 g fiber

430 mg sodium

1. In a large nonstick skillet, heat 1 teaspoon of the oil over medium heat. Place 2 slices of the bread in the pan and top with one-quarter of the cheese and half of the turkey. Spread half of the sauce over the turkey and top with another quarter of the cheese and slice of bread. Cook until browned, for about 4 minutes. Remove from the pan, add another teaspoon of the oil, and cook the second side until toasted, for about 3 minutes.
2. Repeat for the remaining 2 sandwiches.

SUPERFOOD: CRANBERRIES

Cranberries' cheery hue and tart taste wake up muffins, add zing to pork, and make a seriously healthy sandwich spread. Cranberries also, famously, help maintain urinary tract health and are a good source of vitamin C and fiber. You'll get 20 percent of the daily requirement for vitamin C in 1 cup of chopped cranberries.

Fresh, they last 2 to 4 weeks in the fridge and up to a year in the freezer (store in their original packaging or a resealable plastic bag). Grab them October through December, when they're available.

BEEF WITH BROCCOLI, BELL PEPPER, AND MUSHROOMS

PER SERVING:

286 CAL

23 g protein

22 g carbohydrates

12 g fat

3.5 g saturated fat

4 g fiber

787 mg sodium

MAKES 4 SERVINGS

1 tablespoon reduced-sodium soy sauce

1 tablespoon dry sherry

2 teaspoons cornstarch

1 teaspoon sugar

$\frac{3}{4}$ pound flank steak, halved lengthwise, and cut against the grain into $\frac{1}{4}$"-thick slices

1 tablespoon + 1 teaspoon canola oil

4 cups broccoli florets

1 red bell pepper, sliced in $\frac{1}{4}$"-wide strips

6 ounces shiitake mushrooms, stemmed, caps sliced

3 scallions, chopped (white and green parts separated)

1 tablespoon finely chopped fresh ginger

1 tablespoon minced fresh garlic

$\frac{1}{8}$–$\frac{1}{4}$ teaspoon crushed red-pepper flakes

$\frac{1}{4}$ cup water

Classic Stir-Fry Sauce (see below)

1. In a medium bowl, combine the soy sauce, sherry, cornstarch, and sugar. Stir in the beef and set aside for about 15 minutes.
2. Heat a large nonstick skillet or wok over medium-high heat. Add 1 teaspoon of the oil. Swirl to coat. Add half of the beef in a single layer and leave until seared, for about 1 minute. Stir the beef constantly for about 1 minute, until no longer pink. Remove. Add 1 teaspoon of the oil and repeat with the remaining beef.
3. Add the remaining 2 teaspoons of oil to the pan. Add the broccoli, bell pepper, and mushrooms. Stir constantly for 2 minutes. Make a well in the center and add the white part of the scallions, ginger, garlic, and red-pepper flakes. Stir constantly with the vegetables for 1 minute. Add the water and cover the pan until the broccoli is just done, for about 3 minutes. If cooking in a wok, use a large lid, setting it right down into the wok, if necessary, to cover and steam the vegetables.

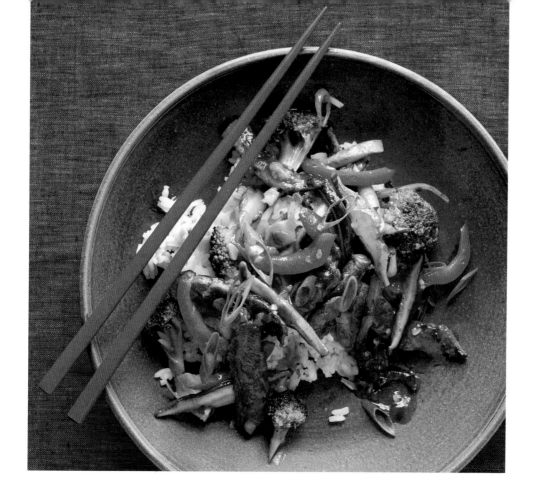

4. Return the beef to the pan and add the Classic Stir-Fry Sauce. Cook until the sauce thickens slightly, for 1 to 2 minutes. Sprinkle with the scallion greens and serve.

Classic Stir-Fry Sauce

Whisk 2 teaspoons of cornstarch into $\frac{1}{2}$ cup of fat-free, reduced-sodium chicken broth (we used Kitchen Basics), and then add 2 tablespoons of oyster sauce, 2 tablespoons of reduced-sodium soy sauce, 2 teaspoons of sherry, and 2 teaspoons of sugar.

GRILLED STEAK WITH AVOCADO

PER SERVING:
395 CAL

28 g protein
30 g carbohydrates
19 g fat
5 g saturated fat
7 g fiber
549 mg sodium

MAKES 4 SERVINGS

- 1 pound flank steak
- 1 lime, halved
- 2 cloves garlic, crushed
- 1 tablespoon ground cumin
- $\frac{1}{2}$ teaspoon ground red pepper
- $\frac{1}{2}$ teaspoon + $\frac{1}{8}$ teaspoon salt
- 8 corn tortillas (6" diameter)
- 1 ripe avocado, peeled and cubed
- $\frac{1}{2}$ cup jarred salsa verde
- 1 scallion, sliced
- 2 tablespoons chopped fresh cilantro

1. Place the steak in a baking dish. Squeeze half of the lime over 1 side of steak and rub with half of the garlic. Sprinkle $\frac{1}{2}$ tablespoon of cumin, $\frac{1}{4}$ teaspoon of red pepper, and $\frac{1}{4}$ teaspoon of salt over the steak. Turn the steak and repeat with $\frac{1}{4}$ teaspoon salt and the remaining lime, garlic, cumin, and red pepper. Let stand for 15 minutes at room temperature.
2. Coat a grill rack with cooking spray. Preheat the grill to medium-high.
3. Grill the steak to the desired doneness, about 4 minutes a side for medium-rare. Transfer the steak to a cutting board and let stand for 5 minutes.
4. Warm the tortillas in the microwave oven.
5. In a small bowl, stir together the avocado, salsa verde, scallion, cilantro, and remaining $\frac{1}{8}$ teaspoon of salt. Cut the steak into thin strips. Serve with the sauce and tortillas.

STEAK CHOICES

Flank, hanger, and skirt steak are butcher favorites because they have a beefier taste than more expensive cuts. Sliced thin, they're tender, too. Any of the three will work here.

BEEF CARNITAS

MAKES 6 SERVINGS

2 pounds lean beef stew meat, cut into $\frac{1}{2}$" pieces

$\frac{3}{4}$ cup mild salsa

2 tablespoons chopped chipotle chili peppers in adobo sauce

$\frac{1}{2}$ teaspoon salt

$\frac{1}{8}$ teaspoon freshly ground black pepper

1 cup beef broth (we used Kitchen Basics) or water

In a large slow cooker, combine beef, salsa, peppers, salt, pepper, and broth. Cover and cook on low for 6 to 8 hours.

PER SERVING:
231 CAL

30 g protein

2 g carbohydrates

11 g fat

4 g saturated fat

1 g fiber

519 mg sodium

MAPLE-LEMON SKIRT STEAK

PER SERVING:

230 CAL

24 g protein	
11 g carbohydrates	
9 g fat	
4 g saturated fat	
0 g fiber	
398 mg sodium	

MAKES 4 SERVINGS

  3 tablespoons maple syrup

  2 tablespoons lemon juice

  1 teaspoon Dijon mustard

  1 clove garlic, minced

  1 pound skirt steak

  $\frac{1}{2}$ teaspoon salt

  $\frac{1}{4}$ teaspoon freshly ground black pepper

1. In a small saucepan, whisk together the maple syrup, lemon juice, mustard, and garlic.

2. Season the steak with the salt and pepper and set aside.

3. Lightly oil a grill pan or heavy skillet and heat over medium-high heat. Cook the steak to the desired doneness, about 3 minutes per side for medium-rare. Transfer to a cutting board and let rest for 5 minutes.

4. Meanwhile, bring the maple-lemon mixture to a boil over medium-high heat. Let simmer for 1 minute. Cut the steak into thin slices across the grain and drizzle with the sauce.

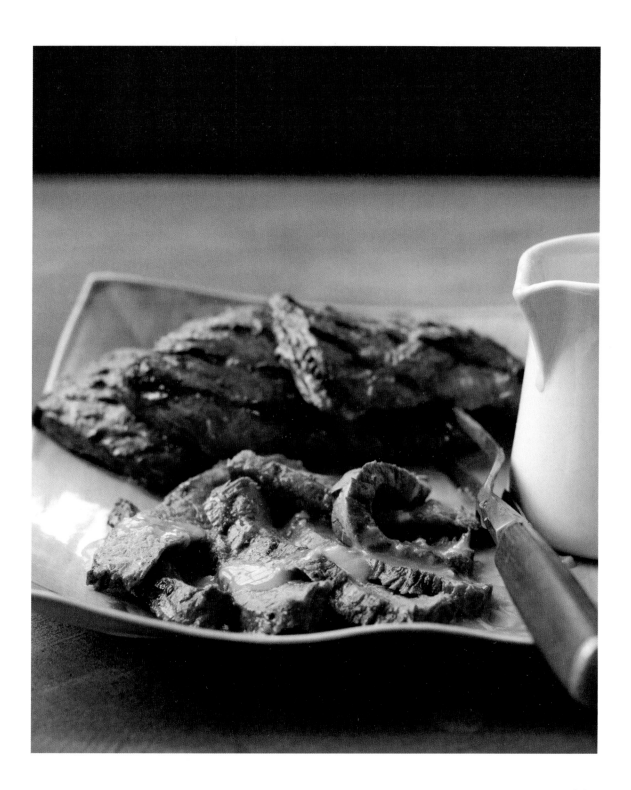

MEAT

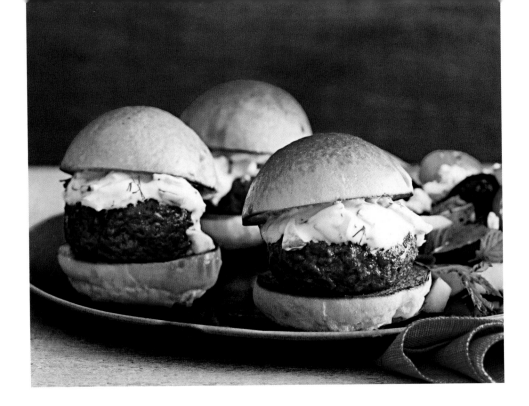

GREEK-STYLE SLIDERS

PER SERVING:

321 CAL

28 g protein

26 g
carbohydrates

12 g fat

4 g
saturated fat

3 g fiber

899 mg sodium

MAKES 4 SERVINGS

1 pound lean ground beef or ground lamb

3 tablespoons tzatziki (we used Cedar's) + additional for garnish

2 teaspoons Greek seasoning blend (we used McCormick)

1/2 teaspoon salt

Pinch of freshly ground black pepper

Party-size potato rolls or dinner rolls (we used Martin's)

1. In a large bowl, combine the beef or lamb, tzatziki, seasoning blend, salt, and a few grinds of black pepper. Shape into 12 miniburgers, about 2" wide.

2. Heat a nonstick skillet over medium heat. Cook the burgers for 3 to 4 minutes, turning once, or until desired doneness. Transfer to sliced buns and spoon a dollop of tzatziki over each burger.

CRANBERRY CHOPS

MAKES 4 SERVINGS

1¼ pounds thin boneless pork chops

½ teaspoon salt

1 teaspoon dried sage (optional)

2 teaspoons vegetable oil

1 clove garlic, minced

¼ cup white wine

½ cup water

1 cup cranberries, chopped

2 tablespoons honey

1 tablespoon whole grain mustard

PER SERVING:
278 CAL

31 g protein

14 g carbohydrates

9 g fat

2 g saturated fat

1 g fiber

408 mg sodium

1. Sprinkle the pork with the salt and sage (if using).
2. In a nonstick skillet, heat 1 teaspoon of the oil over high heat and brown the pork, for 2 to 3 minutes a side. Remove and place the pork on a platter. Lower the heat to medium-low. Add the garlic and cook for 1 minute. Add the wine and scrape up any brown bits. Stir in the water, cranberries, honey, and mustard and simmer until thickened, for about 7 minutes. Spoon over the pork.

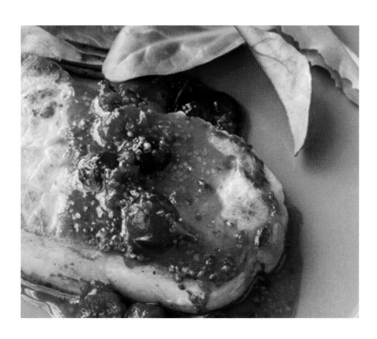

GRILLED PORK AND PLUMS

PER SERVING:
312 CAL

24 g protein

19 g
carbohydrates

16 g fat

5 g
saturated fat

2 g fiber

498 mg sodium

MAKES 4 SERVINGS

- 1 tablespoon finely chopped fresh thyme or 1 teaspoon dried
- ¾ teaspoon ground allspice
- ¾ teaspoon salt
- 4 bone-in, center-cut pork chops (6–7 ounces each)
- 4 red plums (about 1½ pounds total), halved and pitted
- 1 tablespoon extra virgin olive oil

1. In a large bowl, combine the thyme, allspice, and salt. Sprinkle 1 tablespoon of the mixture evenly over both sides of the pork and set aside. Add the plums and oil to the remaining thyme mixture. Let both the pork and plums stand for 15 minutes at room temperature.
2. Coat a grill rack with cooking spray. Preheat the grill to medium.
3. Put the plums on the rack and cook for 5 minutes. Add the pork and grill, turning the pork once, until the plums are tender and the pork is browned on both sides and just cooked through, for 5 to 7 minutes longer.

Simple Swaps

Substitute peaches or nectarines for plums; just grill them a little longer, 10 to 15 minutes. No allspice? Use ¼ teaspoon cinnamon, ¼ teaspoon nutmeg, and a big pinch of ground cloves.

PULLED PORK

MAKES 12 SERVINGS

- 1 teaspoon salt
- 1 teaspoon paprika
- 1 teaspoon chili powder
- ½ teaspoon ground cumin
- ⅛ teaspoon ground red pepper
- 4 pound bone-in pork shoulder, cut into 3 pieces and trimmed of all visible fat
- 1 onion, thinly sliced
- ½ cup brown sugar
- ½ cup ketchup
- ⅓ cup cider vinegar
- ¼ cup tomato paste
- ¼ cup water
- 2 tablespoons mustard
- 2 tablespoons Worcestershire sauce
- ½ teaspoon hot-pepper sauce

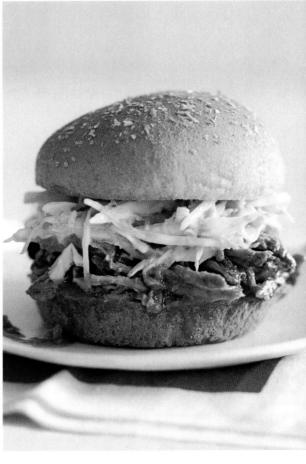

1. In a bowl, mix the salt, paprika, chili powder, cumin, and ground red pepper. Rub all over the pork.
2. In a large slow cooker, combine the pork, onion, brown sugar, ketchup, vinegar, tomato paste, water, mustard, Worcestershire sauce, and hot-pepper sauce. Cover and cook on low for 6 to 8 hours.
3. Remove the pork from the slow cooker and discard the bone. Cool for 10 minutes. Using forks, shred the pork. In a large bowl, combine with the sauce from the cooker.

PER SERVING:
232 CAL

17 g protein	
14 g carbohydrates	
12 g fat	
4 g saturated fat	
1 g fiber	
446 mg sodium	

CORNED BEEF AND CABBAGE

PER SERVING:

322 CAL

| 18 g protein |
| 23 g carbohydrates |
| 17 g fat |
| 5.5 g saturated fat |
| 4 g fiber |
| 1,004 mg sodium |

MAKES 8 SERVINGS

1¼ pounds small red-skinned potatoes, halved

3 medium carrots, peeled and cut into 2" pieces

2 cloves garlic

1 tablespoon brown sugar

1 bay leaf

2½-3 pound corned beef brisket

3 cups water

1 bottle (12 ounces) dark beer

1 small green cabbage, cut into 8 wedges

1. In a large slow cooker, combine the potatoes, carrots, garlic, sugar, and bay leaf. Put the brisket on top of the vegetables and add the water and beer. Cover and cook on low for 8 to 10 hours. Add the cabbage for the last 1½ hours.

2. Remove the brisket from the slow cooker. Let rest, loosely covered, for 5 to 10 minutes before slicing. Remove and discard the bay leaf. Remove the vegetables with a slotted spoon and serve with the brisket.

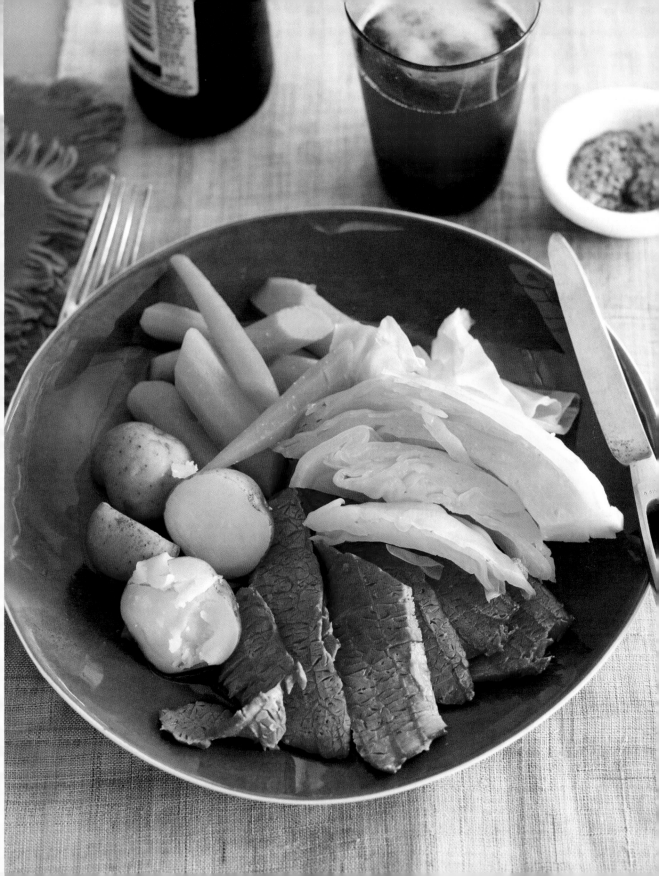

SALMON WITH NOODLES

PER SERVING:
496 CAL

30 g protein
36 g carbohydrates
25 g fat
8 g saturated fat
2 g fiber
697 mg sodium

MAKES 4 SERVINGS

- 4 pieces skinless salmon (4 ounces each)
- 1 teaspoon salt
- 1/4 teaspoon freshly ground black pepper
- 8 ounces egg noodles
- Fresh lemon zest
- 2 tablespoons freshly squeezed lemon juice
- 2 tablespoons butter
- 1 teaspoon extra virgin olive oil
- 1 1/2 teaspoons poppy seeds

1. Preheat the oven to 450°F. Coat a rimmed baking sheet with cooking spray.
2. Season the salmon with 1/2 teaspoon of the salt and 1/8 teaspoon of the pepper. Put the salmon, skin side down, on the prepared baking sheet and bake for 12 to 15 minutes.
3. Meanwhile, prepare the noodles according to the package directions. Drain and toss with the lemon zest and 2 tablespoons of juice from the lemon, butter, oil, poppy seeds, the remaining 1/2 teaspoon of salt, and the remaining 1/8 teaspoon of black pepper.
4. Divide the noodles among 4 plates. Top each with a piece of salmon.

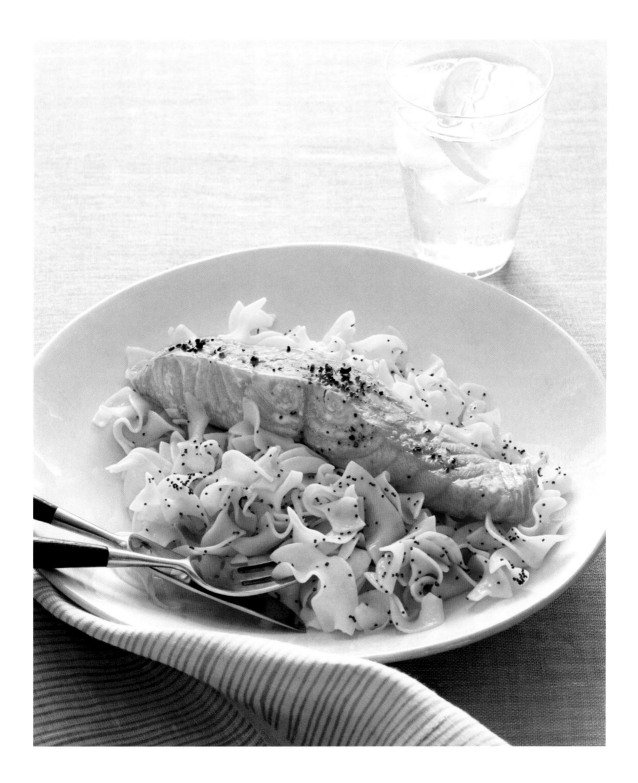

SEARED TUNA WITH TOMATOES AND ARUGULA

PER SERVING:
201 CAL

28 g protein
8 g carbohydrates
6 g fat
1.5 g saturated fat
2 g fiber
204 mg sodium

MAKES 4 SERVINGS

- 2 tuna steaks (about 8 ounces each), each cut in half
- ¼ teaspoon salt
- ¼ teaspoon freshly ground black pepper
- 1 large onion, cut into wedges
- 2 cloves garlic, chopped
- 1 cup halved cherry tomatoes
- 2 tablespoons balsamic vinegar
- 1 bag (5 ounces) baby arugula

1. Sprinkle the tuna with the salt and pepper.
2. Coat a large nonstick skillet with cooking spray and heat over medium-high heat. Add the tuna and cook for 6 minutes, turning once, or until just opaque. Remove to a plate and keep warm.
3. Recoat the skillet with cooking spray. Cook the onion and garlic over medium-high heat for 4 minutes, or until lightly browned. Add the tomatoes and vinegar and cook for 3 minutes.
4. Divide the arugula among 4 plates. Top each with a tuna steak and the tomato mixture.

TUNA CAKES

MAKES 8 SERVINGS

2 cans (12 ounces each) water-packed tuna, drained
1 slice whole wheat bread, toasted and finely chopped
2 tablespoons finely chopped jarred roasted red bell pepper
2 scallions, finely chopped
1 egg, beaten
1 tablespoon mayonnaise
1½ teaspoons lemon-pepper seasoning

PER SERVING:

113 CAL

17 g protein

2 g
carbohydrates

3 g fat

1 g
saturated fat

0 g fiber

368 mg sodium

1. Preheat the oven to 350°F. Coat a baking sheet with cooking spray.
2. In a medium bowl, combine the tuna, bread, pepper, scallions, egg, mayonnaise, and seasoning. With 2 forks, toss the mixture, breaking up the large chunks of tuna, to blend well. With clean hands, shape into 8 cakes. Place on the prepared baking sheet.
3. Bake for 18 to 20 minutes, or until the cakes are golden and heated through.

SEARED SNAPPER ON HERBED MASHED EDAMAME

PER SERVING:

279 CAL

43 g protein

11 g
carbohydrates

5 g fat

0.5 g
saturated fat

4 g fiber

434 mg sodium

MAKES 4 SERVINGS

1½ cups water

2 cups frozen shelled edamame

4 shallots, finely chopped

½ teaspoon dried tarragon

1 tablespoon freshly squeezed lemon juice

1½ pounds snapper, cod, or haddock fillets, cut into 4 pieces

½ teaspoon salt

½ teaspoon freshly ground black pepper

1. In a small saucepan, bring the water, edamame, shallots, and tarragon to a boil over high heat. Reduce the heat to low, cover, and simmer for 20 minutes, or until very tender. Transfer the mixture to a blender or food processor. Blend or process until smooth, adding the lemon juice and a little water if dry. Return to the saucepan, cover, and keep warm.

2. Sprinkle the fish with the salt and pepper.

3. Coat a large nonstick skillet with cooking spray and heat over medium-high heat. Add the fish and cook, turning once, for 8 to 10 minutes, or until the fish flakes easily.

4. Divide the edamame mixture onto 4 plates. Top each with a piece of fish.

STEAMED TILAPIA WITH PESTO

MAKES 4 SERVINGS

PER SERVING:
256 CAL

37 g protein

6 g
carbohydrates

10 g fat

2.5 g
saturated fat

2 g fiber

560 mg sodium

  6 cups fresh baby spinach

  1 red bell pepper, thinly sliced

  4 tilapia fillets (6 ounces each)

$\frac{1}{2}$ teaspoon salt

$\frac{1}{4}$ teaspoon freshly ground black pepper

  4 tablespoons pesto

1. Preheat the oven to 450°F. Coat one side of four 12″ × 20″ sheets of foil with cooking spray.
2. Top half of each foil sheet with 1½ cups of the spinach, one-quarter of the bell pepper, and 1 tilapia fillet. Sprinkle with the salt and black pepper. Fold the other half of each foil sheet over the filling and crimp the edges to make a tight seal.
3. Arrange the packets on a large baking sheet. Bake for 10 to 12 minutes, or until the packets are puffed. Transfer each packet to a serving plate. Carefully slit the top of each to allow the steam to escape. After a minute, peel back the foil to reveal the fish. Check to make sure the fish flakes easily when tested with a fork.
4. Top each portion with 1 tablespoon of pesto before serving.

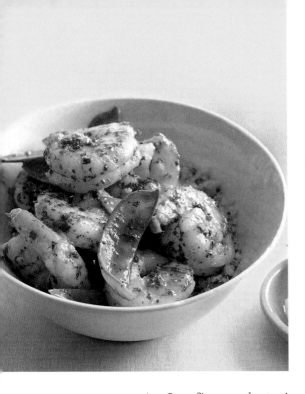

PESTO SHRIMP WITH SNOW PEAS OVER QUINOA

MAKES 4 SERVINGS

¾ cup uncooked quinoa

1⅓ cups water

1 tablespoon olive oil

2 cloves garlic, minced

1 pound large peeled shrimp

3 cups snow peas (about 8 ounces)

¼ cup prepared basil pesto

2 tablespoons lemon juice

PER SERVING:
372 CAL

32 g protein

28 g carbohydrates

15 g fat

3 g saturated fat

4 g fiber

293 mg sodium

1. In a fine mesh strainer, place the quinoa and rinse well under cold water. Transfer the quinoa to a medium saucepan and add the water. Bring to a boil, reduce the heat to low, cover, and simmer until the water is absorbed and the quinoa is tender, for 12 to 15 minutes. Fluff with a fork and cover until ready to serve.

2. Meanwhile, in a large nonstick skillet, heat the oil over medium-high heat. Add the garlic and cook, stirring, for 30 seconds. Add the shrimp and cook, stirring often, until just pink, for about 3 minutes. Stir in the snow peas and cook, stirring, for 2 minutes longer. Add the pesto and lemon juice and cook until warmed and shrimp is done, for about 1 minute. Serve over the quinoa.

EXPERT TIP

For quicker meals, cut out the cutting! Use no-prep produce, such as prewashed spinach, grape tomatoes, and snow peas. Just toss into a pan with a fast-cooking protein and dinner's done.

SPICY SHRIMP MARINARA WITH FETA

MAKES 4 SERVINGS

2	teaspoons olive oil
1	tablespoon minced fresh garlic
¼	teaspoon crushed red-pepper flakes
2	tablespoons white wine
1½	cups jarred marinara sauce
1	teaspoon dried oregano
1	pound large shrimp, peeled
2	ounces feta cheese (about ½ cup)
1	tablespoon chopped parsley

PER SERVING:
242 CAL

27 g protein

11 g
carbohydrates

9 g fat

3 g
saturated fat

2 g fiber

714 mg sodium

1. Preheat the oven to 400°F.
2. In a large ovenproof pan or Dutch oven, heat the oil over medium heat. Add the garlic and red-pepper flakes. Stir for 30 seconds. Add the wine and stir until almost evaporated. Add the sauce and oregano. Let simmer for 5 minutes. Stir in the shrimp. Crumble the feta over top. Bake until the shrimp are just cooked through, for about 8 minutes. Sprinkle with the parsley.

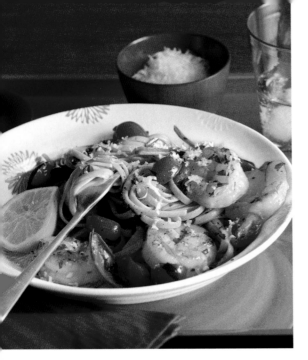

SHRIMP SCAMPI LINGUINE

MAKES 4 SERVINGS

8	ounces whole wheat linguine
1	tablespoon extra virgin olive oil
1	pound medium shrimp, peeled
4	cloves garlic, minced
1/2	teaspoon red-pepper flakes
1	pint cherry tomatoes, halved
1/2	cup dry white wine
	Juice of 1 lemon
1/2	teaspoon salt
3	cups packed fresh baby spinach leaves
1/4	cup finely chopped parsley
1/2	cup grated Parmesan cheese

PER SERVING:

457 CAL

38 g protein

45 g
carbohydrates

12 g fat

3 g
saturated fat

10 g fiber

663 mg sodium

1. Prepare the pasta according to the package directions.
2. In a large skillet, heat the oil over medium heat while the pasta cooks. Add the shrimp, garlic, and red-pepper flakes and cook until the shrimp start to turn pink, for about 2 minutes.
3. Add the tomatoes, wine, lemon juice, and salt. Cook until the tomatoes start to soften, for about 1 minute. Add the spinach and parsley and cook until the spinach wilts, for about 1 minute.
4. Drain the pasta and add to the pan. Toss to coat and serve sprinkled with the cheese.

SEARED CARIBBEAN SCALLOPS WITH BLACK BEAN SALSA

MAKES 4 SERVINGS

PER SERVING:
223 CAL

18 g protein

22 g carbohydrates

8 g fat

1 g saturated fat

5 g fiber

516 mg sodium

- 12 sea scallops (1 ounce each), preferably dry caught
- 1 teaspoon Caribbean jerk seasoning
- 1 can (14.5 ounces) no-salt-added black beans, rinsed and drained
- 1 medium tomato, chopped
- ¾ cup chopped red bell pepper (about 1 medium)
- ½ medium red onion, finely chopped
- 1 small jalapeño pepper, finely chopped (wear plastic gloves when handling)
- 1 cup cubed mango
- ¼ teaspoon ground cumin
- 1 tablespoon chopped cilantro
- 2 tablespoons lime juice
- 2 tablespoons canola oil
- ⅛ teaspoon salt
- Freshly ground black pepper
- 4 lime wedges

1. Place the scallops on a work surface. Pat dry. Dust with the jerk seasoning and toss to coat evenly. Set aside.
2. *To make the salsa:* In a medium bowl, combine the beans, tomato, bell pepper, onion, jalapeño pepper, mango, cumin, cilantro, lime juice, 1 tablespoon of the oil, and salt and pepper to taste, mixing well to combine. Let stand to blend flavors.
3. Meanwhile, heat a skillet over medium-high heat. Add the remaining 1 tablespoon oil and heat for 1 minute. Add the scallops to the skillet. Cook for 1 to 2 minutes on each side, until well browned all over and opaque in the center. Remove to a plate.
4. Spoon the salsa onto 4 dinner plates. Top with the scallops. Place a lime wedge on each plate.

COCONUT ALMOND MACAROONS

PER COOKIE:

32 CAL

| 1 g protein |
| 2 g carbohydrates |
| 3 g fat |
| 1 g saturated fat |
| 1 g fiber |
| 5 mg sodium |

MAKES 52 COOKIES

1½ cups blanched almonds

4 egg whites

1½ cups Splenda Sugar Blend for Baking

1 cup unsweetened coconut

½ teaspoon vanilla extract

1. Preheat the oven to 300°F. Line a baking sheet with parchment paper.
2. Pulse the almonds in a food processor for 15 to 30 seconds, or until finely chopped. Beat the egg whites, using an electric mixer on medium speed for 2 minutes, or until stiff.
3. Gradually fold the Splenda and the almonds into the egg whites. Fold in the coconut and the vanilla.
4. Drop teaspoonfuls of the mixture onto the prepared baking sheet, placing the cookies about 1" apart. Bake for 17 minutes.

WALNUT-PUMPKIN CHEESECAKE

MAKES 8 SERVINGS

- 1 cup 1% cottage cheese
- 8 ounces fat-free cream cheese
- 3 eggs
- ½ cup pumpkin puree
- ⅓ cup + 2 tablespoons maple syrup
- 2 teaspoons pure vanilla extract
- ½ teaspoon ground cinnamon
- ¼ teaspoon ground cloves
- ¼ teaspoon ground fresh ginger
- ½ cup walnuts

PER SERVING:
181 CAL

12 g protein

18 g
carbohydrates

7 g fat

4 g
saturated fat

1 g fiber

341 mg sodium

1. Preheat the oven to 350°F. Coat the bottom and sides of a 9" pie plate with cooking spray.
2. In a blender or food processor, place the cottage cheese. Blend or process for 3 minutes, or until very smooth, scraping down the sides. Add the cream cheese, eggs, pumpkin, ⅓ cup maple syrup, vanilla, cinnamon, cloves, and ginger. Process until very smooth. Pour into the prepared pie plate.
3. Bake for 40 minutes, or until the center is set and a knife inserted in the center comes out clean. Cool completely on a wire rack. Refrigerate for 3 hours or overnight.
4. Meanwhile, coat a small baking sheet with cooking spray.
5. In a small bowl, combine the walnuts and remaining 2 tablespoons maple syrup. Place on the prepared baking sheet. After removing the cake from the oven, bake the nuts for 10 minutes, or until lightly browned. Remove from the oven and let cool on a rack.
6. To serve, arrange the nuts around the edges of the cheesecake.

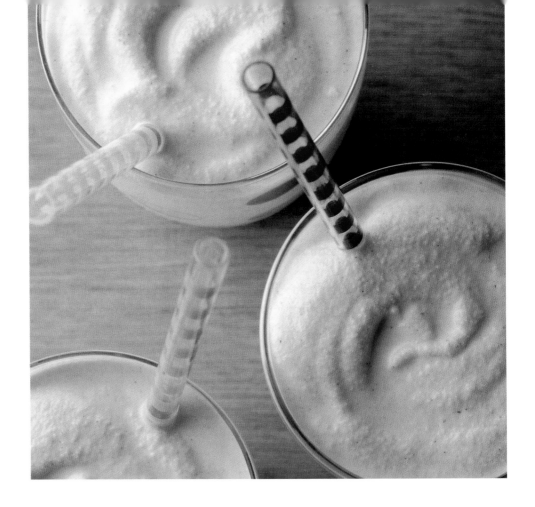

CHOCOLATE-PEANUT BUTTER SHAKE

MAKES 2 SERVINGS

1½ cups cold chocolate soy milk

1 teaspoon vanilla extract

1 small banana

3 tablespoons creamy peanut butter

10 ice cubes

1. In a blender, combine the milk, vanilla extract, banana, peanut butter, and ice cubes.
2. Process until thick and smooth.

CHAI LATTE FRAPPÉ

MAKES 1 SERVING

- 1 chai-flavored tea bag
- ¼ cup boiling water
- ½ cup fat-free vanilla Greek yogurt
- 1 tablespoon ground flaxseed

PER SERVING:
128 CAL

13 g protein	
13 g carbohydrates	
3 g fat	
0.5 g saturated fat	
2 g fiber	
48 mg sodium	

1. Prepare the tea using the water. Let steep for 5 minutes. Discard the tea bag and place the tea in the freezer to chill for 10 minutes.
2. In a blender, combine the tea, yogurt, and flaxseed and pulse until blended. Serve immediately.

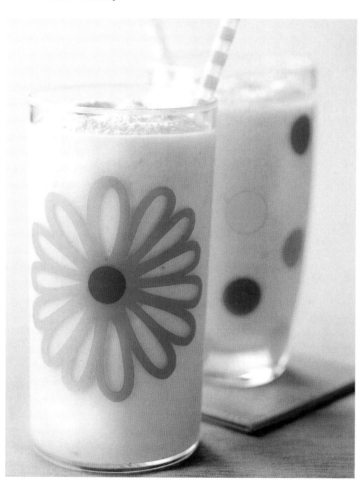

PHOTO CREDITS

INDEX

Boldface page references indicate illustrations. <u>Underscored</u> references indicate tables or boxed text.